END-OF-LIFE
CARE CONSIDERATIONS
for the
SPEECH-LANGUAGE
PATHOLOGIST

Medical Speech-Language Pathology

Series Editors
Kristie A. Spencer, PhD, CCC-SLP
Jacqueline Daniels, MA, CCC-SLP, CBIS

Medical Setting Considerations for the Speech-Language Pathologist
Kristie A. Spencer, PhD, CCC-SLP and Jacqueline Daniels, MA, CCC-SLP, CBIS

Primary Progressive Aphasia and Other Frontotemporal Dementias
Rene L. Utianski, PhD, CCC-SLP

Person-Centered Memory and Communication Interventions for Dementia:
A Case Study Approach
Ellen M. Hickey, PhD, SLP-Reg., SLP(C), CCC-SLP and
Natalie F. Douglas, PhD, CCC-SLP

Tracheostomy and Ventilator Dependence in Adults and Children:
Learning Through Case Studies
Roxann Diez Gross, PhD, CCC-SLP, F-ASHA and Kristin A. King, PhD, CCC-SLP

End-of-Life Care Considerations for the Speech-Language Pathologist
Helen Sharp, PhD, CCC-SLP and Amanda Stead, PhD, CCC-SLP, CHSE

END-OF-LIFE
CARE CONSIDERATIONS
for the
SPEECH-LANGUAGE
PATHOLOGIST

Helen Sharp, PhD, CCC-SLP
Amanda Stead, PhD, CCC-SLP, CHSE

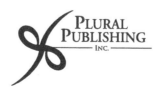

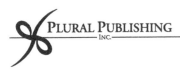

9177 Aero Drive, Suite B
San Diego, CA 92123

email: information@pluralpublishing.com
website: https://www.pluralpublishing.com

Typeset in 11/13 Adobe Garamond by Flanagan's Publishing Services, Inc.
Printed in the United States of America by Integrated Books International

Library of Congress Cataloging-in-Publication Data:
Names: Sharp, Helen (Clinical speech-language pathologist) editor. | Stead,
    Amanda, editor.
Title: End-of-life care considerations for the speech-language pathologist
    / [edited by] Helen Sharp, Amanda Stead.
Other titles: Medical speech-language pathology (Series)
Description: San Diego, CA : Plural Publishing, Inc., [2024] | Series:
    Medical speech-language pathology | Includes bibliographical references
    and index.
Identifiers: LCCN 2023035377 (print) | LCCN 2023035378 (ebook) | ISBN
    9781635506402 (paperback) | ISBN 1635506409 (paperback) | ISBN
    9781635503333 (ebook)
Subjects: MESH: Terminal Care | Speech Disorders—therapy
Classification: LCC RC424.7 .E525 2024 (print) | LCC RC424.7 (ebook) |
    NLM WV 501 | DDC 616.85/5029—dc23/eng/20231121
LC record available at https://lccn.loc.gov/2023035377
LC ebook record available at https://lccn.loc.gov/2023035378

NOTICE TO THE READER
Care has been taken to confirm the accuracy of the indications, procedures, drug dosages, and diagnosis and remediation protocols presented in this book and to ensure that they conform to the practices of the general medical and health services communities. However, the authors, editors, and publisher are not responsible for errors or omissions or for any consequences from application of the information in this book and make no warranty, expressed or implied, with respect to the currency, completeness, or accuracy of the contents of the publication. The diagnostic and remediation protocols and the medications described do not necessarily have specific approval by the Food and Drug Administration for use in the disorders and/or diseases and dosages for which they are recommended. Application of this information in a particular situation remains the professional responsibility of the practitioner. Because standards of practice and usage change, it is the responsibility of the practitioner to keep abreast of revised recommendations, dosages, and procedures.

Contents

Series Introduction

The Medical Speech-Language Pathology book series provides graduate students, clinicians, and clinical researchers with functional, comprehensive material to enhance practice in a medical setting. The books are designed to bolster transdisciplinary knowledge through infusion of information from neurology, pharmacology, radiology, otolaryngology, and other related disciplines. They capture our current understanding of complex clinical populations and offer expert guidance related to evaluation and management strategies. For each book, case studies are used to promote application and integration of the material, and are richly supplemented with figures/photographs and clinical resources. Each book in the series is authored by experienced professionals and content experts who are able to transform the research literature into clinically digestible information, allowing immediate application to everyday practice. This book series advances the medical speech-language pathology community by merging fundamental concepts, clinical strategies, and current theories with research evidence, with the goal of fostering outstanding clinical practice and clinical research.

The **first book** of the series set the stage regarding the environment of the medical SLP as an interprofessional team member, the clinical populations encountered by the SLP, and the foundational knowledge needed to understand and interpret neuroimaging, medication influences, and infection control precautions. The **second book** of the series is an invaluable resource on the frontotemporal dementias (FTDs), including primary progressive aphasia and apraxia of speech. It is a cutting-edge tutorial that encompasses differential diagnosis, clinical examinations, speech/language/cognitive assessments, neuro-imaging findings, and treatment recommendations, with rich supplementary videos and images in the PluralPlus companion website. In the **third book** of the series, the authors harnessed their extensive clinical and research experience with people with dementia, and created a thought-provoking, practical resource. Centering their approach on dignity and empowerment, the authors reframe the traditional clinical approach, and use clinical cases to highlight the fusion of evidence-based practice with culturally responsive care. Clinical guidance is effectively enhanced by materials on the PluralPlus companion website, including photos, forms, and screening tools. The **fourth book** of the series is an innovative and masterful resource on tracheostomy and ventilator dependence. Using 38 real-world case examples across the lifespan, the authors expertly guide us through the complex clinical decision-making process. Case summaries are appropriately contextualized with foundational information and current evidence, and thoughtfully enriched with ample photographs, figures, and supplementary resources.

In this much-anticipated **fifth book** of the Medical SLP book series, Drs. Helen Sharp and Amanda Stead help speech-language pathologists navigate the complex and sensitive issues related to end-of-life care. Based on their extensive experience, the authors coach clinicians through assessment considerations, practical goal setting, and therapeutic options across communication, cognition, and swallowing. They provide expert guidance on ways to enhance positive outcomes while maintaining a focus on humility, and elevating the dignity and autonomy of the patient with a life-limiting diagnosis. With rich resources, including sample scripts, case examples, and clinical decision trees, they empower SLPs to serve as advocates for meaningful end-of-life care. Thoughtful discussions around interprofessional collaborations and practice standards inform the SLP about their roles and responsibilities in this journey with the family. This exceptional book will undoubtedly become a valuable resource for SLPs as well as students and course instructors. Through the lens of compassion, it serves as a thoughtful guide for SLPs to honor the choices of the pediatric and adult clients with life-limiting conditions.

Medical Speech-Language Pathology
Series Editors
Kristie A. Spencer, PhD, CCC-SLP
Jacqueline Daniels, MA, CCC-SLP, CBIS

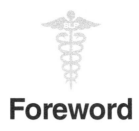

Foreword

This long-needed compendium of information and advice about end-of-life care should give speech-language pathologists (SLPs) the confidence to offer skilled services to patients with terminal conditions who have difficulty communicating. As the recent COVID-19 pandemic painfully highlighted, the communication needs of individuals at the end of their life are more complex than having someone's hand to hold or seeing familiar faces on a computer screen. Many SLPs experienced frustration at being overlooked when the medical team was focused on patients' medical needs without full consideration of the importance of communication to patients' well-being. Our collective years of experience providing creative solutions to the communication challenges of adults with aphasia, ALS, and dementia and children with cystic fibrosis, cancer, and other disorders have armed us with a variety of tools to serve the unique needs of these populations. The contributors to this book have shared their insights and experiences about how to determine the conditions for optimum sensory input and the support needed for clear expression of thoughts and emotions. They provide specific examples of how to have difficult conversations, how to determine patient capacity for decision making, and how to write goals for meaningful interactions that promote the best possible quality of life during the dying process.

The adage "with age comes wisdom" may resonate with many SLPs who have practiced for 20 to 30 years. We have learned through experience, and trial and error, how to address the challenges presented by our patients as we thought, "I never learned about this in school." As young clinicians, most of us were enthralled with the possibilities of helping our clients learn to communicate better and to reach their communication goals. It was not until we encountered patients who were terminally ill that we realized we might not know what to do to support their communication needs at the end of life.

My own "aha" moment came 15 years ago at my grandmother's funeral when the chaplain of her nursing home explained that we were about to experience a memorial service developed through conversations they had had with my grandmother in the last few months of her life. The prayers and songs of the service were my grandmother's favorites, but no one in the family would have known this. Many of our last conversations with her were to encourage her to "fight the good fight" and to "keep walking and eating to stay strong." It occurred to me that this chaplain had given my grandmother and our family a great gift—a meaningful way to say goodbye. She could do this because she was not family, fraught with emotion about our grandmother's imminent passing. The chaplain was able to be a neutral and empathetic person who could ask the difficult questions, offer support, and obtain objective responses.

I realized that SLPs could and should be the neutral person to discuss important topics with patients who are terminally ill. But without specific training in how to do this, it is unlikely that SLPs, especially those newest to clinical practice, would feel capable of expanding their scope of practice in this way. SLPs need to be prepared to help patients and their families communicate about important topics at the end of life. This textbook provides practical and useful guidance for effective practices that allow patients to embrace quality of life until the very end.

Michelle S. Bourgeois, PhD, CCC-SLP
Tampa, FL

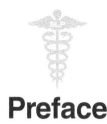

Preface

One of the essential qualities of the clinician is interest in humanity, for the secret of the care of the patient is in caring for the patient.

—F. W. Peabody, 1927

The purpose of this book is to cultivate an understanding of the value of caring for patients with life-limiting conditions and for anyone facing their final weeks or days of life. For speech-language pathologists (SLPs), the idea of working with patients who do not have an expectation of recovery is too often perceived as fundamentally different from the (re)habilitation work an SLP usually does. However, the SLP's core knowledge and skills in speech, voice, language, cognition, communication modalities, eating, drinking, and swallowing places us as essential service providers for patients in decline. The fundamental shift for SLPs is to adopt a palliative care approach that holds quality of life, symptom management, and the patient's goals of care at the center (Pollens, 2012). Our goal in developing this book is to empower SLPs to serve as advocates who support the rights and needs of people with life-limiting conditions to eat and to communicate from the time of diagnosis through end of life.

Throughout the book we discuss *life-limiting conditions* to encompass any serious and incurable health condition. Decline in health is a process that may take years, months, or days. The *end-of-life* period generally reflects a likelihood of death within the foreseeable future, usually months, weeks, or days. Regardless of where a patient is on the trajectory toward death, at no time is it futile for a patient to communicate with their loved ones or to convey symptoms or other care needs to their health care providers.

Woven through the book is a core theme highlighting the essential role of humility for clinicians who work with patients with life-limiting conditions and those nearing the end of life. While each chapter presents common elements of care that emerge in clinical practice, the unique needs of each patient and family are of utmost importance. We use the term "humility" with deliberate acknowledgment of the work of Tervalon and Murray-Garcia (1998), who coined the term "cultural humility" to embody a commitment to lifelong learning and self-reflection, attention to the power imbalances between clinicians and patients, the importance of active listening, and true shared decision making with patients. Each of the components of cultural humility applies to every aspect of caring for patients in every context and is of utmost importance when we have the privilege of supporting people through their final days.

One example of a way in which clinicians can embody humility is to avoid assumptions about the patient's lived experience. An example of this is to avoid the use of the phrase "suffers from" in clinical notes or case examples. We often see notes that begin with a phrase such as "Joaquim suffers from multiple sclerosis. . . . " This phrase is not grounded in the patient's perspective, but rather assigns suffering to the patient from the perspective of the clinician. Instead, clinical writing can and should simply state "Joaquim is diagnosed with multiple sclerosis . . . " or " . . . has multiple sclerosis." If the individual clearly conveys suffering through what they say or how they respond, then the clinician should report this observation, ideally using the words of the patient in a direct quote.

Although many SLPs find themselves working with individuals who do not have a pathway to recovery or cure, very few training programs address the role of the SLP in palliative and end-of-life care (Pascoe et al., 2018). This book is designed to introduce practicing SLPs and students who plan to become SLPs to the many ways in which their knowledge and skills can improve the lives of patients and their families as they face declining health and the trajectory toward death.

We recognize that training curricula are already dense with requirements, so we have designed this book so that individual chapters can be incorporated into existing coursework. We have also included teaching resources (Appendix A) to support faculty, instructors, and guest speakers with materials and examples to support the integration of palliative and end-of-life care in coursework. The activities and learning outcomes are designed to support a unit within a course such as aphasia, dysphagia, augmentative and alternative communication (AAC), counseling, interprofessional education, or professional issues. The book and instructional resources also provide a solid foundation on which to build a freestanding seminar or course in end-of-life care.

We are beyond grateful to the clinician–scholars who contributed their knowledge and experience to this book. Although social norms cast death and dying as "gloomy" topics to be avoided, in each chapter the authors have deftly captured the importance, joys, and fulfillment of clinical work with individuals who have life-limiting conditions. Each author concurrently

recognizes the essential need for interprofessional team care for the benefit of patients and caregivers and as a mechanism for clinicians to manage the heaviness of this work. Every chapter includes practical tips, sample scripts, case examples, and practical advice grounded in the clinical experiences of the chapter authors. The authors collaborated, exchanged ideas, and brought the full depth of their knowledge and clinical experiences to this book with the hope that their words will inspire you to serve patients with life-limiting conditions.

REFERENCES

Pascoe, A., Breen, L. J., & Cocks, N. (2018). What is needed to prepare speech pathologists to work in adult palliative care? *International Journal of Communication Disorders*, *53*(3), 542–549.

Pollens, R. (2012). Integrating speech-language pathology services in palliative end-of-life care. *Topics in Language Disorders*, *32*(2), 137–148.

Tervalon, M., & Murray-Garcia, J. (1998). Cultural humility versus cultural competence: A critical distinction in defining physician training outcomes in multicultural education. *Journal of Health Care for the Poor and Underserved*, *9*(2), 117–125.

All names used in scripts and case examples are fictitious and all cases have been modified to protect patient privacy.

Contributors

Riwa Al Aridi, PharmD
Faculty of Pharmacy
Lebanese International University
Beirut, Lebanon
Licensed Pharmacist
Walgreens
The Villages, Florida
Chapter 1

Michelle S. Bourgeois, PhD, CCC-SLP
Professor, Retired
University of South Florida
National Aphasia Association
Primary Progressive Aphasia Task Force
Tampa, Florida
Foreword, Chapter 4, and Appendix B

John Costello, MA, CCC-SLP
Director
Augmentative Communication Program
    and Jay S. Fishman ALS Augmentative
    Communication Program
Boston Children's Hospital
Boston, Massachusetts
Chapter 6

Julieta Gilson, MD, FACP
Assistant Professor
University of Central Florida
Orlando, Florida
Palliative and Hospice Medicine
Naples Community Hospital
Naples, Florida
Chapter 1

Marnie Kershner, CScD, CCC-SLP, BCS-S, CBIS
Senior Inpatient Speech-Language
    Pathologist
MedStar National Rehabilitation Hospital
Washington, D.C.
Chapter 5

Paula Leslie, PhD, FRCSLT (U.K.), Reg HCPC (U.K.), CCC-SLP
Affiliated Faculty
Center for Bioethics & Health Law–
    Research Ethics & Society Initiative
University of Pittsburgh
Pittsburgh, Pennsylvania
Chapter 5

Robin Pollens, MS, CCC-SLP
Coordinator and Clinical Supervisor
Aphasia Communication Enhancement
    Program
Adjunct Professor
Department of Speech, Language, and
    Hearing Sciences
Western Michigan University
Kalamazoo, Michigan
Chapter 2

Rachel M. Santiago, MS, CCC-SLP
Clinical Coordinator and Speech-Language
    Pathologist
Inpatient Augmentative Communication
    Program
Boston Children's Hospital
Boston, Massachusetts
Chapter 6

Helen Sharp, PhD, CCC-SLP
Research Facilitator,
Interdisciplinary Research Lab in Palliative
    and End-of-Life Care
University of British Columbia Okanagan
    Kelowna, British Columbia
Chapters 2, 3, and Appendix C

Joseph W. Shega, MD
Executive Vice President and Chief Medical
    Officer
VITAS Healthcare

Associate Professor of Medicine
University of Central Florida
Gotha, Florida
Chapter 1

Amanda Stead, PhD, CCC-SLP, CHSE
Professor, School of Communication
   Sciences and Disorders
Pacific University
Forest Grove, Oregon
Chapters 2, 4, and Appendices A and B

Rami Tarabay, MD
Associate Medical Director
VITAS Healthcare
Clermont, Florida
Chapter 1

Jordan R. Tinsley, MS, CCC-SLP
Clinical Assistant Professor
Communication Sciences and Disorders
Pacific University
Forest Grove, Oregon
Appendix A

To our patients and our students.
You are our best teachers.

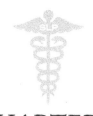

CHAPTER 1

Introduction to End-of-Life Care for the SLP

Joseph W. Shega, Rami Tarabay, Riwa Al Aridi, and Julieta Gilson

> *"To cure sometimes, to relieve often, and to comfort always."*[1]

INTRODUCTION TO HOSPICE AND PALLIATIVE CARE

Palliative care and hospice represent a continuum of health care services for persons with serious illness from the time of diagnosis of a medical condition through death and bereavement care (Figure 1–1). Balfour Mount is credited with coining the term "palliative care," which is derived from the Latin root word "pallium," which refers to a cloak or outer garment. The term palliative reflects care that cloaks or covers the symptoms of serious illness. Palliative care has been defined in several ways over time, with more recent emphasis on caring for persons with serious illness. Kelley and Bollens-Lund (2018) defined serious illness as a "health condition that carries a high risk of mortality and either negatively impacts a person's daily functioning or quality of life or excessively strains his or her caregiver" (p. S-8). Table 1–1 summarizes the terminology incorporated into definitions of palliative care from leading organizations in palliative medicine and health care, including the American Academy of Hospice and Palliative Medicine (AAHPM), Center to Advance Palliative Care (CAPC), National Consensus Project (NCP), and the World Health Organization (WHO).

Palliative care emphasizes both patient and family, with a focus on improving quality of life through the assessment and management of pain and other symptoms, achievement of the patient's goals and preferences, and coordination of care across disciplines and settings. This comprehensive approach to care addresses physical, psychological, social, and spiritual domains through an interdisciplinary team that includes a speech-language pathologist (SLP). Palliative care can be incorporated

---

[1]Source unknown but attribution in the literature includes Hippocrates, a 15th-century folk saying, Sir William Osler, Edward Livingston Trudeau, and others. Often used by the hospice movement to highlight the importance of the role of care, even when a cure cannot be achieved.

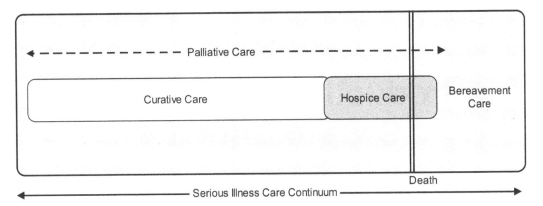

Figure 1–1. The continuum of care from time of diagnosis through death. Palliative care focuses on symptom management and quality of living with a serious illness. Hospice care is a type of palliative care offered to patients as they near the end of life. Hospice care encompasses care for the patient in the context of their family and close friends with services that extend beyond the patient's death.

at any time in the trajectory of illness, with earlier adoption as the standard of care.

Hospice is a type of palliative care and is implemented as patients approach the end of life (EoL). The term "hospice" is derived from the Latin word "hospis," meaning hosts and guests, the same root word that yields "hospital" and "hospitality." Hospice represents a service delivery system that incorporates the philosophies and approaches to palliative care with an emphasis on helping the patient transition from life to death and explicitly addresses the care of the family and other personal caregivers. A key component of hospice is to offer care in the community and in a location that the patient calls home, which can include a nursing home or assisted living.

In the United States, hospice is a defined insurance-covered benefit for someone who has a prognosis of life expectancy of 6 months or less if the illness runs its normal course. Hospice care coverage mandates specific components as part of the care model and provides a fixed rate of reimbursement for each day of care (Greenstein et al., 2019). This fixed rate (or capitated payment) covers all care related to the patient's terminal prognosis and is not adjusted for acuity or complexity of the care

provided. Under United States guidelines, hospice services must also provide bereavement services for the family after the death without additional reimbursement. To access hospice care, a patient or their proxy must elect to enroll and consent to a care plan that is palliative, not curative, with an emphasis on quality of life. At any time, a patient or family can revoke the hospice benefit and resume access to traditional medical care.

Hospice care is delivered by a core interdisciplinary team that includes a physician, nurse, social worker, chaplain, home health aide, bereavement counselors, and volunteers. Other disciplines are incorporated in the patient's care as needed to achieve the palliative care plan. Other skilled services may include dietary, pharmacy, physical and/or occupational therapy, and speech-language pathology. Home medical equipment and medications are covered by the hospice program.

Patients benefit from the availability of four levels of care—(1) routine, (2) inpatient, (3) continuous, and (4) respite—with each level of care designed to keep patients in their preferred location. Confusion often exists around continuous care, which is only

Table 1–1. Language Incorporated in Commonly Used Definitions of Palliative Care

Source	Focus	Goals	Domains	Time Frame	Other
American Academy of Hospice and Palliative Medicine	Patient Family	• Quality of life • Treat disease-related distress	• Physical • Intellectual • Emotional • Social • Spiritual	Any stage of illness	• Autonomy and choice • Preferred therapies • Appropriate anytime and location
Center to Advance Palliative Care (consumer definition)	Patient Family	• Relief from the symptoms and stress of an illness • Quality of life	• Not addressed	Based on need, not prognosis	• Any age or stage • Provided along with curative treatments • Extra layer of support: Physicians, nurses, and other specialists
National Consensus Project	Patient Family	• Assessment and management of pain and other symptoms • Support of caregiver needs • Coordination of care • Assess preferences and how to achieve them	• Physical • Functional • Psychological • Practical • Spiritual	Appropriate at any stage of illness, ideally early integration in care plan	• Interdisciplinary • Offered in all care settings
World Health Organization	Patient Family	• Quality of life patient and caregiver • Relieve suffering through assessment and management of pain and other problems	• Physical • Psychological • Social • Spiritual	Life-threatening illness	• Team approach • Bereavement counseling • Human right to health • Needs and preferences of the individual

employed when a patient develops uncontrollable symptoms from an exacerbation or disease progression and incorporates a nurse or home health aide to be in the home to support a patient and family up to 24 hours a day. However, hospice does not provide nonskilled or custodial in-home care. Routine custodial care is expected to be provided by family members or by assistants a family may choose to hire. Families may be eligible for respite care, which refers to short-term (5 consecutive days) inpatient support designed to support rest and recovery for family caregivers.

Hospice services and, to a lesser extent, palliative care services, have been demonstrated in multiple studies to improve the quality of patient care at a reduced cost (Aldridge et al., 2022; Kleinpell et al., 2019). Family caregivers for hospice recipients report better pain and symptom management, increased likelihood of emotional support, sense of respect through service delivery, and overall improved satisfaction with care when compared with reports from caregivers whose family members died without hospice services (Kleinpell et al., 2019; Teno et al., 2004). At the same time, hospice care substantially decreases the likelihood of hospitalization and emergency department use without adversely impacting life expectancy, with total cost of care also significantly lower for those who receive hospice services (Kelley et al., 2013).

THE ROLE OF REHABILITATION AND RESTORATIVE CARE IN PALLIATIVE CARE

In general, the overall goal of rehabilitation and restorative care is to help patients regain physical abilities with a focus on independence. Interventions are designed to optimize function and reduce disability from health conditions and their interaction with the environment (Balen et al., 2019; Dahl,

2002). Such interventions benefit from self-management skills, adaptive equipment, rehabilitation (self-care, mobility, and functional independence), and chronic disease management. Despite the most robust interventions, patients near the EoL typically fail to benefit from such an approach and may experience worse quality of life and other health care outcomes (e.g., increased hospitalizations, emergency room visits, and health care costs). Of significance to outcomes, when services focus on maximizing function, patients and families may lose the opportunity to complete other critical life tasks such as achieving a life goal, saying goodbye to loved ones, or managing personal affairs.

Care plans that focus on palliation and quality of life frequently derive substantial benefit from therapy services that traditionally focus on rehabilitation. For example, physical therapy may be able to restore sufficient mobility to optimize ease of transfers from chair to bed or to achieve safe and efficient ways to turn a loved one to avoid painful pressure sores and to change bed linens. Similarly, speech-language pathology services can contribute substantively to a palliative and EoL care plan in a variety of impactful ways. For example, compensatory strategies that help patients maintain oral intake for as long as possible or access to alternative communication strategies enable a patient to express their needs more effectively and to participate in goals of care conversations with physicians and other team members. With these impacts in mind, hospice programs in the United States are required to provide access to therapy services that include physical, occupational, and speech-language pathology services.

Persons with serious illness often have distinct yet overlapping goals that at times may seem to conflict with one another. For example, a patient may simultaneously want to live as long as possible, be as strong as possible, be at home, and optimize quality of life despite a progressive illness with a life expectancy of weeks. While medical care teams strive to achieve all patient goals, in some cases tradeoffs must occur and are delineated through the process of shared decision making to reach agreed-upon goals of care. Such conversations help identify the type and intensity of health care services a given patient may opt to receive. Clear goal-setting is particularly important as many services may be available simultaneously but focus on and cover very different care plans.

Differentiating Therapy Services by Setting

Three commonly available services for persons with serious illness in the United States include skilled nursing facility care (surrounding a hospitalization), home health, and hospice services. Some of the key differences in characteristics are shown in Table 1–2. Skilled nursing facility services and home health may incorporate palliative care outside of an insurance or Medicare hospice benefit, but these services are not typically as comprehensive or structured to meet the specific, complex, and rapidly evolving needs of patients who are dying. Although there is certainly overlap, in general, skilled nursing facility services and home health generally focus on restorative care, whereas hospice focuses on supportive services with treatment decisions tailored and limited to those that enhance the patient's quality of life.

FACTS AND FIGURES: PALLIATIVE CARE AND HOSPICE SERVICES IN THE UNITED STATES

America's Care of Serious Illness 2019 State-by-State Report Card reported that at least 12 million adults and 400,000 children have a serious illness such as cancer, heart disease, renal disease, or dementia (Morrison & Meier, 2019). It is expected that the majority of the large "baby boomer" population (those born between 1946 and 1964) will experience a chronic illness over the next decade.

To help meet the need for palliative care, the number of hospital-based palliative care teams continues to increase. Among hospitals with 50 or more beds, 72% report a palliative care team in 2019, which is a sizeable increase from 67% in 2015 and 7% in 2001. The larger the hospital, the more likely a palliative care team exists, with 94% of hospitals with more than 300 beds reporting a palliative care team, in contrast to 62% of hospitals with 50 to 299 beds (Morrison & Meier, 2019). Rural hospitals are substantially less likely have access to palliative care, with just 17% versus 90% of urban areas with 50 or more beds (Morrison & Meier, 2019). Outpatient and community-based palliative care programs continue to increase in number but are generally limited in access due to barriers to insurance coverage and scalability.

In comparison, access to hospice care is almost universal for adults in the United States because it is a defined benefit covered by most insurers and approximately 80% to 90% of those enrolled through Medicare. According to National Hospice and Palliative Care Organization (NHPCO) statistics, 1.61 million Medicare beneficiaries who died in 2019, or 51.6% of all Medicare decedents, were enrolled in hospice care for 1 day or more (NHPCO, 2021). In general, referral to hospice occurs relatively late in the course of disease and hospice lengths of stay tend to be short. A Medicare hospice benefit defined as a prognosis of 6 months or less has an 18-day median length of service and mean length of hospice of 93 days (NHPCO, 2021).

Hospice use increases with age, and by age 85 and older almost 63% of Medicare decedents are enrolled under the hospice benefit. Despite increased use rates, significant health

Table 1–2. Care Options Available Near the End of Life in the United States

Characteristic	Skilled Nursing Facility	Home Health	Hospice
Eligibility	Qualifying hospital stay 3 consecutive midnights Skilled need: therapy services or nursing 24-hour nursing care in a facility	Face-to-face physician visit within 90 days to establish need with certification every 60 days Skilled need: therapy services or nursing Homebound except for short durations of time	Physician-certified prognosis <6 months, if disease runs normal course Palliative not curative care plan Not required to be homebound
Duration of services	1–20 days full coverage; 21–100 days partial coverage with coinsurance; >100 days no coverage Must meet the skilled need and make progress toward a goal	Limited number of visits based upon diagnosis Must document progress within the length of service allowed	Unlimited number of visits based on patient need and care plan
Location	Inpatient	Community	Community, assisted living, long-term care
Payment	Medicare Part A	Medicare Part A	Medicare Part A
PT/OT/Speech	Restorative	Restorative/functional	Functional/palliative
Palliative care	Infrequent	Infrequent	Always
Medications	Yes	No	Yes
Equipment	Yes	No	Yes
After-hours staff availability	Yes	No	Yes
Physician available	Yes	No	Yes
Bereavement	No	No	Yes

disparities are evident in hospice utilization statistics, with 54% of White Medicare beneficiaries, 43% of Hispanic Medicare beneficiaries, 41% of Black Medicare beneficiaries, and 38% of Asian American and American Indian/Alaska Native Medicare beneficiaries who died while enrolled in hospice (NHPCO, 2021).

ESTABLISHING GOALS OF CARE

The field of medicine generally focuses on the diagnosis and management of diseases, with little incorporation of patient preferences or priority-aligned decision making that considers individualized goals of care. This is particularly relevant in palliative care and hospice, as serious illness studies document that the health care patients experience is often not consistent with their values (Khandelwal et al., 2017). Patients' health status influences the intensity and focus of health care, with the relative emphasis on patients' wishes and values increasing as life expectancy decreases and as the focus of care shifts from hospital-based cure or restorative goals to quality of life or palliative goals of care. Research with patients nearing the EoL finds that patient's goals include individual preferences for care (e.g., being at home), pain and symptom management, emotional well-being, being treated with dignity, clinical adherence to treatment preferences, and time with loved ones (Meier et al., 2016). Engaging in care goal conversations over time facilitates a patient-centric approach that integrates the patient's values, wishes, and priorities in the context of medically appropriate treatment through shared decision making (see also Chapter 3).

Differentiating Goals of Care From Advance Care Planning

One common area of confusion is the difference between "goals of care" conversations that focus on current and ongoing medical decisions and "advance care planning" that serves as the care plan should the patient not be able to make decisions for themselves. For example, advance care planning can lead to the creation of an advance directive that outlines the care one would want when diagnosed with a life-limiting condition and the inability to communicate one's wishes (e.g., living will), the appointment of a health care power of attorney to make health care decisions should one become unable, and wishes related to cardiopulmonary resuscitation. Although goals of care conversations may focus on advance

care planning, the primary goal of goals of care discussions are to clarify what patients and their families value most and to facilitate the creation of a care plan to support those goals.

A goals of care conversation aims to support informed decisions based on the patient's values and preferences. Goals of care may focus on the benefits and risks of any of the following areas of decision making:

- the approach of care, such as skilled care with intensive rehabilitation versus hospice with palliative-driven interventions
- the location of service delivery (role of hospitalization or intensive care unit [ICU] care versus care delivery at home with hospice support)
- decision making about whether to continue current nonpalliative therapies such as a ventilator, chemotherapy, or any other treatment or medication regimen
- decision making about prospective or proposed assessments and treatments, such as a new chemotherapy or initiating dialysis

As the care team discusses the patient's preferences and undesired side effects or other burdens of treatment, it is critical to provide clear guidance that if certain treatments are stopped (or not started), the intensity that surrounds *care* is never stopped.

A patient and family may express multiple goals that they want to be met concurrently but are not possible to achieve simultaneously. Such apparent conflicts may create uncertainty for clinicians about how to incorporate the patient's goals into a feasible care plan. In these circumstances, clinicians provide ongoing support and clear communication to help the patient identify their priorities. Through counseling and discussion, clinicians work to support patient understanding that certain goals may need to be sacrificed to meet other goals with a higher priority.

Clinicians should continuously revisit patients' goals because preferences and goals often change with experience of disease and disability. Although these changes are expected, at times these shifts may seem sudden and it may be difficult for the patient and family to adapt, particularly when health changes unexpectedly for the worse. Despite these challenges, studies document that clinicians skilled in communication can help patients and families navigate serious illness and EoL discussions without adverse mental health consequences. Moreover, such conversations lead to improved quality of life, better patient and family satisfaction, increased completion of advance directives, less unwanted and nonbeneficial care, and reduced health care costs (Wright et al., 2008).

Many clinicians feel unprepared and uncomfortable initiating goals of care conversations. It is important for all clinicians to develop skills in having necessary conversations about health, illness, and EoL. Approaches to break down these barriers and improve communication skills include:

- Complete training courses in communication and elucidation of care goals
- Incorporate a standardized approach to having the conversation
- Identify colleagues with expertise in your practice setting and shadow their goals of care conversations
- Engage in conversations with patients and families with reflection upon what went well and areas to improve with the next encounter

Table 1–3 details examples of standardized approaches to goals of care conversations.

Table 1–3. Models for Systematic Approaches to Difficult Conversations to Support Breaking Bad News and Developing Goals of Care

Approach	Brief Description
SPIKES; Baile et al., 2000	**S**et up the interview **P**erception of the patient **I**nvitation obtained **K**nowledge and share information **E**motion and empathetic responses **S**trategy and summarize
REMAP; Childers et al., 2017	**R**eframe **E**xpect emotion **M**ap the future **A**lign with patient values **P**lan treatment
SUPER; Pollak et al., 2019	**S**etup **U**nderstanding **P**riorities **E**xplain **R**eview and recommend

The Role of the Speech-Language Pathologist in Goals of Care Discussions

SLPs have a critical role within the context of goals of care conversations. Communication often becomes impaired in serious illness, so an SLP can help leverage communication strategies to optimize the patient's ability to understand and to express their goals and values. The inclusion of adaptive equipment to support patient care may include call buttons or other environmental control switches, communication boards, speaking valves for patients with tracheostomy tubes, or electronic communication systems. Improvements in communication help patients engage in these important conversations and offer the opportunity for more meaningful and impactful discourse with their loved ones (see also Chapters 2, 4, and 6).

An SLP can also elucidate preferences related to eating as a social function. This includes the sensory experience of eating along with establishing the patient's preference for management approaches to swallowing difficulties, such as conversations around the utility, safety, and burdens of the use of thickening products (Wang et al., 2016). Discussions with the medical team, patient, and caregivers about the use of artificially administered nutrition and hydration and alternatives to tube feeding, such as careful hand feeding and comfort feeding, similarly benefit from SLP participation (see also Chapter 5).

Goals of care around swallowing issues may incorporate the SLP to help delineate whether to pursue a restorative/functional or a functional/palliative care plan. A key component to that conversation is the medical history and the status of medical conditions that can impact swallowing with the incorporation of the results of swallowing studies. The SLP can help develop strategies to manage dysphagia symptoms and work with the patient and family to not only optimize feeding strategies for comfort and eating satisfaction, but also help the medical team identify the best approach to medication formulations for symptom management. For example, pills can be difficult to swallow, but if the patient is able to swallow liquids, physicians and pharmacists may modify the formulation for a given medication to allow for ease of oral delivery or to deliver the medication nonorally. A number of medications can be delivered sublingually and do not rely on swallowing skills.

Taken together, the SLP has a key role to help delineate goals of care and to support patients and families with serious illness through EoL by serving as a key expert on the interdisciplinary team to improve communication strategies and to optimize swallowing support, including management of dysphagia symptoms that cause discomfort. These contributions are paramount given that decrements in communication and swallowing are almost universal as part of the dying process.

DEATH AND DYING: CLINICAL PATHWAYS AND APPROACHES TO MANAGEMENT

Natural History of Serious Illness

In general, diseases such as coronary artery disease, heart failure, chronic obstructive pulmonary disease, colon cancer, cerebral atherosclerosis, and other chronic health conditions are the consequence of a significant exposure or susceptibility that triggers subclinical changes that over time lead to the onset of symptoms and a clinical diagnosis. Although these conditions may be treated with optimal medical and behavioral approaches to care, which may slow progression, these progressive diseases often result in declines in health over time. The trajectory of decline varies substantially among individuals based upon the diagnosis itself, timeliness of diagnosis, available treatments, adherence to treatments, comorbid conditions, social determinants of health, and many other factors. Health decline may be seen through nutritional and functional deterioration, progressive increase in symptoms, and/or intermittent exacerbations including hospitalizations and ultimately end-stage disease.

Trajectories of Dying

Three distinct functional decline patterns emerge near the EoL for people with progressive chronic illness: terminal disease, organ failure, and frailty (Lunney et al., 2003). A fourth trajectory, sudden death, is much less common in the developed world and constitutes less than 10% of deaths. Examples of sudden death include cardiac arrest, stroke, aneurysm, or a fall resulting in a brain bleed. Of note, homicide, suicide, substance abuse, and fatal motor vehicle accidents are generally excluded from sudden death estimates and constitute 5% to 6% of deaths in the United States. The understanding and recognition of disease trajectories can help clinicians prognosticate and offer better care for very sick patients and can help patients and their families understand what to expect in their future health.

Terminal Disease Trajectory

The terminal disease trajectory is denoted with steady progression and a clear terminal phase with rapid functional decline several months before death. Patients with cancer diagnoses most commonly follow this trajectory and account for 20% to 30% of all fatalities annually (Lunney et al., 2002).

Functional decline is evident when activities of daily living (ADLs) are monitored. Typically, six ADLs (bathing, dressing, continence, transfers, ambulation, and eating) are tracked. On average, ADL dependency is 0.77 one year prior and 4.09 one month prior to death (Lunney et al., 2003). When substantial decline in functional status occurs, patients also often experience concurrent symptoms such as pain, shortness of breath, anxiety, and depression. Of note, the use of antitumor therapy (immunotherapy, chemotherapy, radiation therapy, or combination of cancer therapies) at this point of disease progression exacerbates symptoms and may shorten life. Given the more distinct terminal phase with substantial observable functional decline over a relatively short period of time, health conditions that follow this trajectory generally have the highest rates of hospice referral and enrollment.

Organ Failure Trajectory

Organ failure accounts for 16% to 30% of all fatalities in the United States, with an average age of death greater than the terminally ill group, but lower than the frailty group, with almost 40% of people who die with organ failure in the range of 75 to 84 years of age. Progressive conditions include heart, lung, liver, kidney, and other renal-related conditions, as well as some neurological diseases.

Progressive conditions often have a prolonged onset and course of illness characterized by gradually deteriorating function and intermittent exacerbations of the underlying condition. Acute illnesses such as infections may also occur and contribute to rapid decline or to a pattern of exacerbation and recovery. Initially, exacerbations may be followed by a full functional recovery, but over time and with disease progression, recovery patterns do not return to previous pre-exacerbation levels. For patients with organ failure, the functional trajectory of the six ADLs at the EoL is 2.10

ADL dependency 1 year prior and 3.66 one month prior to death (Lunney et al., 2003). Patients, families, and clinicians often struggle to determine proximity to EoL due to the inherent unpredictability of the exacerbation–recovery cycle. The impact of this uncertainty yields inconsistent or little access to hospice services or to very late referral for hospice services with a length of stay of often measured in days or weeks.

Frailty Trajectory

The frailty trajectory accounts for 20% to 47% of all deaths and represents the oldest age group, with 66% of deaths occurring among individuals aged 80 years or older. This pathway is common in Alzheimer-type dementia and other dementias, as well as some neurological diagnosis such as Parkinson's disease, multisystem atrophy, and progressive supranuclear palsy.

This patient population is characterized by significant comorbidity and functional disabilities, which result in poorer quality of life over longer periods of time due to the gradual yet progressive decline. Deterioration continues steadily, typically with fewer crises than may be seen in the organ failure trajectory. However, infections, dehydration, falls with fractures, or eating problems may occur over time and eventually lead to the patient's death. The functional trajectory of the six ADLs at the EoL is 3.00 ADL dependency 1 year prior and 5.84 one month prior to death (Lunney et al., 2003). Patients within this risk group often transition to an assisted living or nursing home and often access hospice services for longer periods of time when compared with patients in other trajectory groups.

Active Dying

Active dying or imminent death is the final stage of the dying process. Many terms, defi-

nitions, and accompanying time frames exist, and each represent the stages associated with the last few weeks of life. At this stage, patients experience a number of physiological changes that impact neurocognitive, cardiovascular, pulmonary, and muscular function.

Clinicians should be skillful at identifying this phase because clear communication facilitates patient and family capacity to address personal, social, financial, and medical decision making. When patients and families understand the underlying processes, their satisfaction with care increases and the complexity of the grieving process that follows the patient's death decreases for family members (Teno et al., 2004). Clarity about imminent death allows patients and families to focus on what is important to them, which is often being at home and surrounded by loved ones (Meier et al., 2016). For patients very near the EoL, closure often includes the completion of four key tasks: personal forgiveness, forgiveness of others, expression of thanks, and being able to communicate "I love you."

The first step in the care of a patient who is actively dying is to identify the clinical signs of dying and educate patients and families about what they represent and what to expect as the process evolves. Table 1–4 summarizes common clinical signs of imminent death, the average time of onset before death, a description of a positive clinical sign, and related management approaches. The more clinical signs that are present, the higher the likelihood death will occur within the next couple of days.

Clinicians should also discuss appropriate transitions of care to ensure the patient and family needs can be met at the preferred location with superior outcomes occurring with hospice services alongside family support. Patient and family support are foundational in ongoing education and counseling. Lastly, physical (e.g., pain, shortness of breath, agitation) and nonphysical (e.g., anxiety, depression,

Table 1–4. Clinical Signs of Dying

Clinical Sign	Median Time Onset to Death	Description and Positive Sign	Management Approaches
Peripheral edema	>7 days	Accumulation of fluid resulting in swelling; location is generally most dependent parts of the body such as the arms and legs	• Repositioning • Diuretics
Delirium	>7 days	Poor attention with acute onset and fluctuating course; severe confusion sometimes associated with hallucinations, abnormal drowsiness and/or restlessness, pacing, and agitation	• Evaluate for contributing causes • Reassurance, orientation, eye glasses/hearing aids • Discontinue anticholinergic medications • Antipsychotics
Dysphagla—solid foods	>7 days	New onset difficulty swallowing solids	• Educate • Change food consistency
Decreased speech output	7 days	Less able to communicate through words	• Educate • Adaptive devices, if applicable
Cool/cold extremities	7 days	Skin of legs and then arms feels cold to the touch	• Educate • Blankets
Abnormal vital signs	4–6 days	High heart rate (>100) or respiratory rate (>20) Low systolic (<100) or diastolic (<60) blood pressure	• Educate • Discontinue blood pressure medications
Decreased level of consciousness	5.5 days	Somnolence (sleepiness, drowsy, ready to fall asleep) and/or lethargy (drowsiness where the patient can't be easily awakened)	• Educate
Dysphagia—liquids	5.5 days	Difficulty swallowing liquids	• Educate • Keep mouth moist (wet sponge or oral swab, crushed ice, coating the lips with a lip balm)
Palliative Performance Scale (PPS) 20% or less	3 days	Bedbound, unable to do any work, total care, minimal intake/sips	• Educate
Peripheral cyanosis	3 days	Bluish discoloration of extremities	• Educate

Table 1–4. *continued*

Clinical Sign	Median Time Onset to Death	Description and Positive Sign	Management Approaches
Decreased response to visual stimuli	3 days	Decreased response to visual cues	• Educate
Drooping of the nasolabial fold	2.5 days	Decrease in prominence/ visibility of nasolabial fold (see appendices for pictures)	• Educate
Hyperextension of the neck	2.5 days	Neck becomes hyperextended	• Educate • Opioids if pain present
Cheyne-Stokes breathing	2 days	Alternating periods of apnea and hyperpnea with a crescendo–decrescendo pattern	• Educate • Opioids if dyspnea present
Nonreactive pupils	2 days	Flash light into pupils to see if they react Pupils do not constrict in response to brief exposure to bright light	• Educate
Decreased response to verbal stimuli	2 days	Decreased response to verbal cues	• Educate
Death rattle	1.8 days	Gurgling sound produced on inspiration and/or expiration related to airway secretions	• Educate • Repositioning • Anticholinergics if patient suffering
Apnea	1.8 days	Prolonged pauses between each breath	• Educate • Opioids if dyspnea present
Respiration with mandibular movement	1.8 days	Depression of jaw with inspiration	• Educate
Decreased urine output	1.8 days	Measured volume of urine over a 12-hour period <100 mL	• Educate
Pulselessness of radial artery	1.5 days	Inability to palpate radial pulse	• Educate
Inability to close eyelids	1.5 days	Eyelids do not close	• Educate • Wet washcloth if eyes dry/irritated

continues

Table 1–4. *continued*

Clinical Sign	Median Time Onset to Death	Description and Positive Sign	Management Approaches
Grunting	1.5 days	Sound produced predominantly on expiration, related to vibrations of vocal cords	• Educate • Opioids if pain present
Fever	1.5 days	Temperature >100 F	• Cool washcloth on patient's forehead and removing blankets • Fan • Acetaminophen

spiritual distress, loss of meaning) symptoms should be assessed, monitored, and managed by appropriate members of the care team.

Common Symptoms and Management Approaches as Patients Near Death

The most common symptoms patients experience near the EoL include pain, shortness of breath, anxiety, depression, fatigue, agitation, nausea and vomiting, and constipation. The symptoms a given individual experiences in the trajectory toward death can vary substantially even for the same diagnosis, so individualized, comprehensive, and ongoing assessment remains paramount.

Assessment of symptoms relies on patient self-report, professional and family proxy report, and direct observation. As death approaches, assessments become multifaceted to ensure all symptoms are addressed. When the presence of a given symptom is unclear but suspected, a trial of empiric treatment is often implemented. For example, if a patient cannot communicate pain with a pain scale, other symptoms such as facial grimace, vocalization, or movement will yield a trial of pain management to evaluate if symptoms subside with treatment.

It is beyond the scope of this chapter to detail a comprehensive assessment and management approach of each of the most frequently observed symptoms. However, an overview of common symptoms with accompanying treatments is presented in Table 1–5.

Given that the natural history of dying nearly always includes dysphagia and decreased level of consciousness, medication delivery often has to be modified from oral to alternate routes of administration. Due to the frequency of dysphagia and the likelihood of SLPs consulted related to dysphagia, Table 1–5 emphasizes alternative routes of medication administration. Most often sublingual delivery or transdermal (e.g., patches) are used and if these fail, rectal or parenteral administration are initiated. The overwhelming majority of patients can tolerate sublingual delivery of medication until the time of death (Robison et al., 1995).

Table 1–5. Management of Symptoms Frequently Experienced Near the End-of-Life and Commonly Used Interventions. Example Medications Include Emphasis on Medications that Can be Delivered when Patients Experience Difficulty with Oral Intake.

Symptom	Treatment Type	Examples of Interventions	Special Considerations
Pain	Nondrug Interventions	• Turning • Range of motion • Thermal (heat and cold) • Massage • Transcutaneous electrical nerve stimulation (TENS)	• Often difficult to tolerate with disease progression
	Topical Medications	• Nonsteroidal anti-inflammatory drugs (NSAIDs) cream or gel (e.g., diclofenac) • Local anesthetics (e.g., lidocaine patch)	• Challenge to keep patches in place
	Systemic Medications	• Nonsteroidal anti-inflammatory drugs (NSAIDs) (e.g., ibuprophen) • Analgesics (e.g., acetaminophen liquid) • Opioids—immediate release (e.g., rapid acting fentanyl) • Opioids—short acting (e.g., liquid morphine or hydromorphone) • Opioids—long acting (e.g., liquid methadone, transdermal buprenorphine, transdermal fentanyl)	• NSAIDS and analgesics aid with fever management as well as pain • Rapid release opioid agents are extremely expensive • Not all patients will be candidates for these medications due to drug interactions and metabolic impact • Liquid versions with high concentrations in small volume available • **Do not crush or chew** long-acting formulations
Shortness of breath	Nondrug Interventions	• Repositioning • Oxygen (hypoxia only) • Fans • Guided imagery	• Oxygen no better than room air in the absence of hypoxia • Fans have some evidence of efficacy
	Systemic Medications	• Short and long acting opioids (see pain) • Benzodiazepines (e.g., lorazepam liquid or crushed tablet) • Nebulized albuterol and/or ipratropium	• Benzodiazepines are more effective with concomitant anxiety • Inadequate evidence for use of nebulized opioids • Ipratropium has anticholinergic effects that may impair cognitive function, increase anxiety, or increase insomnia

continues

15

Table 1–5. *continued*

Symptom	Treatment Type	Examples of Interventions	Special Considerations
Anxiety and restlessness	Nondrug Interventions	• Music • Guided imagery • Hypnosis • Mindfulness meditation • Cognitive behavioral therapy	• Many of these interventions are effective, but are not appropriate when patients are actively dying
	Systemic Medications	• Benzodiazepines (e.g., lorazepam liquid or crushed tablet) • Other agents (e.g., trazadone, buspirone, antipsychotics, selective serotonin reuptake inhibitors [SSRIs])	• Long-acting clonazepam effective, but cannot be crushed • "Other" agents rarely used in patients who are actively dying except antipsychotics • Many antipsychotics are available in liquid (haloperidol and risperidone) or can be delivered via intramuscular or intravenous injection (or other parenteral delivery route)
Depression	Nondrug Interventions	• Movement • Cognitive behavioral therapy • Existential psychotherapy (dignity therapy)	• Unclear benefit when initiated at end of life except existential psychotherapy/dignity therapy designed for brief intervention with patients who have a terminal illness
	Systemic Medications	• Reuptake Inhibitors: selective serotonin reuptake inhibitors (SSRIs) & serotonin and norepinephrine reuptake inhibitors (SNRIs) • Tricyclic antidepressants (TCA) (e.g. nortriptyline • Stimulants (e.g., methylphenidate tablet)	• Efficacy at end of life, timeframe is a factor with expectation several weeks of medications for symptom management • Stimulant effects observed usually with days
Fatigue	Nondrug Interventions	• Aerobic and strengthening exercises	• Not generally used in end-of-life care
	Systemic Medications	• Steroids (e.g., prednisone tablet or oral solution, dexamethasone tablet, oral solution or injectable, methylprednisolone depo and intravenous) • Stimulants (e.g., methylphenidate, modafinil armodafinil)	• Stimulants have faster onset of action • Typically short duration of use • Methylphenidate offers best evidence among stimulants

Table 1–5. *continued*

Symptom	Treatment Type	Examples of Interventions	Special Considerations
Delirium with agitation or terminal restlessness	Nondrug Interventions	• Address underlying contributors (e.g., stop use of medications with anticholinergic effects and other contributing medications) • Optimize environment	• For mild to moderate symptoms non-drug interventions are a first-choice intervention • Use of physical restraints should be avoided
	Systemic Medications	• Antipsychotics (e.g., haloperidol tablet via liquid or parenteral, quetiapine tablet) • Benzodiazepines (e.g., lorazepam liquid or crushed tablet)	• Only indicated for severe symptoms • Several of these medications can be crushed or are available in liquid form • Monitor for paradoxical agitation
Nausea or vomiting	Nondrug Interventions	• Avoid strong smells or other triggers • Small frequent meals • Limit oral intake during severe episodes • Relaxation • Aromatherapy (e.g., peppermint, lavender) • Acupuncture and/or acupressure (e.g., wrist bands, P6 stimulation)	• Hunger and oral intake generally decline as death approaches and feeding may exacerbate nausea or vomiting and worsen quality of life
	Systemic Medications	• Dopamine blockade (e.g., haloperidol tablet, liquid, or parenteral delivery; metoclopramide tablet or intravenous; prochlorperazine tablet or rectal) • Selective serotonin receptor (SSR) (5-HT3) antagonists (e.g., ondansetron oral, intravenous, or dissolvable tablet)	• Haloperidol strongest dopamine blocker; usually first line empiric treatment • SSR medications may be very well tolerated and are used with chemotherapy, radiation, and post-operative nausea

continues

Table 1–5. *continued*

Symptom	Treatment Type	Examples of Interventions	Special Considerations
Constipation	Nondrug Interventions	• Movement • Hydration • Discontinue medication with anticholinergic effects	• Dietary bulk forming agents (e.g., fiber) are strongly discouraged
	Systemic Medications	• Osmotic agents (e.g., polyethylene glycol liquid, sorbitol liquid, magnesium sulfate liquid) • Stimulants (e.g., senna tablet and liquid; disacodyl tablet or suppository) • Peripheral μ-Opioid Receptor Antagonists (PAMORA) (e.g., methylnaltrexone bromide subcutaneous; pegylated naloxone tablet)	• Avoid lactulose as it produces gas which causes discomfort • Avoid docusate as it causes mushy stool with no benefit • Opioid receptor agonists only used for refractory opioid related constipation

*For patients who have difficulty eating due to dysphagia or cognitive status, it is essential to verify whether medications can be crushed or given in alternate forms prior to recommending modified administration to the patient or family. Slow release or long-acting medications should not be crushed or administered in forms other than as prescribed.

COUNSELING PATIENTS AND CAREGIVERS

The Value of Excellent Communication Skills

Communication is a core skill that benefits hospice and palliative care health care professionals. In fact, specialists in palliative and hospice care often describe their procedure or medical intervention as the ability to communicate essential and sensitive information to persons with serious illness and their family members. When clinicians overlook emotional, spiritual, and social concerns they may inadvertently exacerbate a patient's suffering by focusing only on the disease. It is essential for clinicians to take time to listen to a patient's life stories and work to understand and honor their meanings, even when clinicians may lack a personal frame of reference or bring a different worldview.

In hospice and palliative care, the three most common elements of communication are transmitting medical information, engaging in therapeutic dialogue, and sharing decision making with patients and their families. Transmitting medical information often involves sharing bad news while engaging in therapeutic dialogue to explore how the patient and family are coping with the illness and attempting to understand their deepest concerns. Shared decision making facilitates the discussion of the patient's values and preferences while benefiting from the clinician's knowledge and expertise to come to a joint decision for care.

Honest and compassionate communication is at the foundation of a trusting clinician–patient relationship. The focus of communication generally shifts as EoL approaches. Initially, the focus of communication is often information giving, but over time and with disease progression, therapeutic dialogue becomes much more important. Patient and family members look to clinicians not only for medical knowledge and technical skill, but also for guidance, reassurance, hope, meaning, and compassionate understanding. The ability to communicate effectively and compassionately is essential as it contributes to the creation and maintenance of a therapeutic relationship, which directly impacts the outcomes for patients, families, and caregivers long after the patient's death.

Effective communication with patients and their caregivers remains the foundation of an optimal clinician–patient relationship and is essential to high-quality person-centered care. Although this is widely known, training programs for health care professionals primarily focus on how to diagnose and treat illness, without adequate attention to communication strategies, especially those that include EoL discussions. The involvement of patients and families in meaningful, sensitive communication represents a critical component of a clinician's responsibility, although studies document that such conversations are generally short or do not occur at all. As described in the Goals of Care section, communication techniques can be taught and practiced using established frameworks (see Table 1–3).

The literature and clinical experience uphold the benefits of effective communication with respect to clinical outcomes for patients and families, health systems, and clinicians. Interventions that enhance clinician communication have been associated with favorable patient outcomes including improved quality of life and mood, improved adherence to treatment regimens, and a preference for less burdensome care as death approaches (Back et al., 2009). Family members also benefit from an improved understanding of patient goals and demonstrate better psychological adjustment and reduced depression and anxiety after the death of their loved one. For the health system, effective communication reduces decision-making conflict and errors, which helps care teams to function more effectively and ultimately mitigates malpractice litigation. When patients and families are included in decision making, length of stay in intensive care units decreases, with an associated reduction in total cost of care for patients who no longer benefit from such an approach (Kyeremanteng et al., 2018). Finally, clinicians benefit from enhanced communication skills, as it has been found to increase empathy and decrease burnout while increasing a sense of personal achievement (Back et al., 2009; Bumb et al., 2017).

Approach to Communication

The first step in effective communication is to identify and overcome cultural, psychological, language, listening, and system-related barriers. Cultural barriers represent the patient and family's essential beliefs and values, or how they relate to the world. This may include expectations of the health care system, the influence of religion and spirituality, personal and societal values about self-worth, lack of experience with death and dying, and/or approach to information disclosures by the clinical team. Psychological barriers incorporate patient and family fears along with the fears of clinicians such as expressing emotion, doing harm, or coping with death. Language barriers may reflect lack of familiarity with medical jargon, underlying language disorders such as aphasia, limited English proficiency, and/or lack of access to interpreters. Barriers to listening may occur for the patient related to limited attention span, noisy or chaotic environment, or hearing loss. System barriers represent a lack of organizational support, reimbursement challenges, adequate time for clinicians to spend with patients, and/or financial, geographic, transportation and/or other barriers to access to appropriate medical care for serious illness.

General strategies for effective communication can improve the quality of conversations, particularly those that are difficult or emotionally charged. As with any new skill, formal or semiformal instruction, deliberate practice, and feedback all improve communication skills for clinical professionals (Back et al., 2009). Effective communication strategies and examples are given in Table 1–6 and can be incorporated as part of ongoing conversations with patients and families when discussing serious illness. Of note, one strategy that must be used with caution, but that can be enormously therapeutic, is the appropriate use of humor. Humor should not ridicule, destroy confidence, or undermine teamwork, but rather should build confidence and connection through shared understanding.

Communicating Serious Illness

The way in which communication of serious illness occurs has a lasting impact on patients and their family members and other caregivers. Difficult conversations are generally not a one-time event, but rather an ongoing process as clinicians often underestimate the amount of information a patient and family want. For example, most patients with a terminal illness know they are dying and the tendency to avoid discussions of prognosis is likely to increase their sense of loneliness and abandonment while denying them opportunities for meaningful communication about death-related issues. However, some patients do not want to know about their diagnosis, prognosis, or treatment options, so it is important to ask patients and families what information they do and do not want to discuss.

There are multiple structured approaches available to assist clinicians as they build core skills in breaking bad news and goals of care conversations (Baile et al., 2000; Childers et al., 2017; Pollak et al., 2019). Each structured approach to conversation about serious illness has common elements (see Table 1–3), including an appropriate physical setting with adequate time to have the conversation with the necessary attendees (e.g., patient and family members). Prior to delivering the news, it is critical to understand what the patient already knows about the illness, which offers a starting point along with insights about how previously shared information has been assimilated. Once the patient's current level of understanding is known, the clinical team asks how much the patient wants to know and subsequently shares information. Prior to discussing serious news, a warning is generally given to prepare the patient and family. This is an iterative process of information sharing and ascertainment of understanding and requires that clinicians respond to emotions, exhibit empathy, and continually assess patient readiness and state to receive and understand the information to be delivered. Finally, next steps are discussed. While this may occur in an initial meeting or in a subsequent one, clinicians should expect to repeat and revisit decisions with patients and their families. Examples of structured approaches to communication are summarized in Table 1–3. Clinicians new to this work should learn one framework and adopt it as part of their clinical practice to ensure difficult news and subsequent care planning is conducted in a comprehensive and consistent way.

One key component of conversations about serious illness is the concept of hope. Over the course of illness progression, hopes generally change from cure to disease control to not wanting to suffer. A common phrase used in hospice and palliative care is, "we hope for the best and prepare for the worst."

Table 1–6. Common Strategies for Effective Communication

Strategy	Examples
Nonverbal cues	• Good eye contact at patient level or lower • Sit close to patient as relationship dictates • Lean toward the patient • Silence to ensure patient and family can share thoughts • Soft touch as warranted by relationship and situation
Empathy	• Remain present even when patient is suffering • Do not always need to "take action" but be in the moment • Elicit, acknowledge, and validate patient feelings • Name the emotion: "You seem angry." • Acknowledge the patient's experience: "I can't possibly understand what you are going through." • Exhibit respect: "I've been so impressed how you have handled this illness. You are doing all the right things." • Show support including nonabandonment: "I will be here for you." • Explore emotions: "Tell me more about what worries you." • "I wish" statements: "I wish we had better treatment options for your [condition]." • Use of the word "we": "I know this is not the result we were hoping for." • Pair hope with worry phrases: "I am hopeful your cancer will respond to the next treatment, but I worry you will not be able to tolerate it because you are so weak."
Open-ended questions	• "How are you doing today?" • "Tell me about your difficulty with eating and drinking." • "Tell me why you seem so distracted." • "How are your loved ones coping with your [condition]?"
Verbal and nonverbal listening responses	• Verbal "Hmm," "Uh-huh," "Oh," "Then," "And" • Nonverbal Eye contact, nodding head, leaning toward the speaker
Repetition	• Repeat one or two words from the last sentence spoke to indicate you are listening; this encourages ongoing dialogue and helps indicate the speaker is being heard
Paraphrasing	• Repeat patient or family sentence in your own words to ensure the message was understood "When you think about dying, you worry about not being able to eat and being hungry?"
Clarifying responses	• "Can you give me an example of what you were talking about?" • "You have talked a lot about when you are feeling well. Can you tell me about when you are not feeling well?" • "In the past how have you coped when you feel overwhelmed?"

continues

Table 1–6. *continued*

Strategy	Examples
Confrontation and honest labeling	• "You say that you are not sad, but whenever we talk about your son, you begin to cry. Can you tell me what you are feeling about your son?" • "You say that everything is okay, but you keep talking about being alone. What is worrying you?"
Summarizing	• "So what I am hearing you say is . . . " • "What I am understanding based on our conversation is . . . "

An important role of the clinician is to help patients and families reframe hope through realistic goals. Another building block of hope is to communicate and demonstrate nonabandonment. Clinicians should always avoid phrases such as "there is nothing more we can do for you" as it is associated with high emotional distress and does not reflect the reality of the situation. Reassurance that the clinician will stay with the patient through this process can be invaluable.

PALLIATIVE CARE AND HOSPICE SERVICE DELIVERY

Service Delivery Models

In the United States, hospice services were foundational with the growth of palliative care based in the successes of the hospice model. Hospice is distinct as it focuses on delivery of care wherever the patient calls home and is a defined benefit reimbursed by Medicare and Medicaid. To be eligible for hospice services, two physicians must agree that the patient has a terminal illness and a life expectancy of 6 months or less. Palliative care grew out of a primary shortcoming of hospice care, namely the need for symptom management for patients who did not qualify for hospice

services together with the needs of hospitalized patients near the EoL who could not benefit from the community-based hospice model and often endured intensive care interventions and substantial suffering up until their death. Hospital-based palliative care programs began because so many seriously ill patients experienced prolonged hospital stays with little or no discussion of symptom burden, care goals, and care options. These programs were paid for by health systems using a fee-for-service framework, recognizing that program revenues did not meet expenses but reduced costs of care while improving patient experience.

Palliative care programs continue to evolve based upon the needs of seriously ill patients and reimbursement mechanisms. With the success of hospital-based initiatives, programs expanded to include outpatient clinics, long-term acute care (LTAC) institutions, and skilled nursing facilities. In these settings, a highly efficient program staffed primarily by advance practice nurses (nurse practitioners) could be offered and be cost neutral given insurance coverage for the service. More community-based programs have subsequently emerged and necessitate more novel reimbursement mechanisms outside of traditional fee-for-service models. An example of alternate reimbursement models is a per-member, per-month payment or risk-based incentive model derived from cost savings associated alternate models of care delivery outside the hospital.

Palliative care service availability continues to expand through health systems or in partnership with hospice programs doing "upstream" care to address patient care needs and facilitate smooth transitions as patients become eligible for hospice. Other specialists that often care for persons with serious illness, namely geriatricians and home-based providers, have also started to add palliative services as part of their care model. Most recently, independent palliative care providers have initiated community-based services, particularly in the context of accountable care organizations or management service organizations that coordinate care for patients enrolled in fee-for-service Medicare and Medicare Advantage, respectively. Telemedicine has served as a catalyst to increase access to community-based palliative care since it offers ease of scale independent of the geographic limitations that often impact scheduling of home-based care and associated labor costs (e.g., urban traffic or rural drive times).

Palliative Care and Hospice Quality

In the United States, hospice has been a defined Medicare and private insurance benefit for more than 40 years after being passed into law because hospice services improved outcomes at lower cost and thus provided value for patients, families, and the health care system. Specifically, hospice beneficiaries had improved health-related outcomes such as better satisfaction with care and pain management, increased likelihood of being treated with respect, having their emotional needs met and EoL needs addressed, and lower psychological distress. These services were achieved at lower cost outside of hospitals and in the patient's preferred location (usually at home). While these and other outcomes have been monitored over time, in recent years these data have become publicly available by providers.

Quality metrics reported for hospice services include process, costs and claims, and patient/caregiver survey data. Process measures represent a composite score reflective of admission procedures. Claims-based outcomes focus on a hospice's use of higher levels of care, costs, the provision of care, and discharges from hospice not due to death. Primary caregivers receive a survey after the death of a loved one with focus on communication, timeliness of care, training, emotional support, and global measures of satisfaction such as whether they would recommend hospice services to others.

Palliative care outcomes remain nascent with no national standards and an evolving landscape of outcome measures that vary by service delivery site, organizational structure, and payer preferences, despite calls from stakeholders to develop outcome metrics. For example, the AAHPM, in conjunction with National Coalition for Hospice and Palliative Care (NCHPC) and the RAND Corporation, developed measures to assess efficacy of pain and symptom management and whether patients felt their preferences were understood. Other organizations advocate for advance care planning and set goals for care systems such as continuity of care (e.g., fewer transitions of care) and location of care (e.g., increased number of days at home). More timely transitions to hospice and hospice length of stay represent important outcomes and can be somewhat captured in a discharge index, which compares deaths of patients receiving palliative care who die with or without hospice services. Finally, accountable care organizations and management service organizations often include measures surrounding utilization such as number of hospitalizations or total cost of care.

THE PALLIATIVE CARE AND HOSPICE TEAM

Interdisciplinary care is the standard of care for hospice service delivery (Greenstein et al., 2019). The composition of the interdisciplinary team varies substantially across hospice and palliative care programs. In the United States, Medicare mandates that the core interdisciplinary team include a physician, nurse, social worker, and pastoral worker with additional team members available when needed such as hospice aides, occupational and physical therapists, SLPs, dieticians, and others (Centers for Medicare and Medicaid Services, 2021). Use of volunteers is also a mandate, and volunteers serve as an important adjunct to the care team. Key members of the interdisciplinary care team and their respective roles are shown in Table 1–7. In contrast to hospice, palliative care service delivered outside of a defined hospice program is highly variable in team composition. Variability is driven by the origins of the program within medical systems, the goals of the program, and by reimbursement models.

Both hospice and palliative care teams work with a patient's primary care team to provide support for people with serious illness. The focus of hospice and palliative care services is to provide relief from physical, psychological, spiritual, and social symptoms and improve quality of life for both the patient and their family.

Palliative care can be provided at any stage of serious illness and is generally provided along with curative-intent treatment, so the components of the team may change over time. For example, at the time of diagnosis, a physician and advance practice nurse may meet the patient's and family's needs through outpatient services, while later in disease progression, nurse and social worker support in the patient's home may be more appropriate until the patient can transition to full hospice services delivered at home or through center-based hospice care.

A key component of the interdisciplinary team is regular interdisciplinary group (IDG) meetings. The purpose of IDG meetings is to conduct a comprehensive discussion of each patient's goals of care and care plan. This approach ensures a cohesive care plan that is updated regularly based upon patient and family needs and facilitates shared understanding across members of the hospice team. In addition to the care team members, some IDGs incorporate the patient and families themselves and may include the patient's primary care clinicians to facilitate care coordination within and among teams.

ACCESS CONSIDERATIONS FOR PALLIATIVE CARE AND HOSPICE

Palliative care programs improve patients' physical and psychological symptom control and quality of life and improve caregiver well-being with reduced stress and dysfunctional grief. At the same time, these services reduce the cost of care or are cost neutral relative to hospitalization costs. Despite significant evidence that seriously ill patients substantively benefit from palliative care, with earlier access generating the greatest benefit, many people living with serious illness either do not receive any palliative care service or receive services only as they are very near the EoL. For example, in the United States, only about 50% of patients die with hospice service support. When hospice services are provided, referral occurs very late in disease trajectory with short lengths of stay. About one-quarter of patients receive hospice services for a week or less and 50% of patients receive services for 30 days or less before death. Barriers to access and timely access to hospice services are recognized worldwide. To address gaps in access,

Table 1–7. Roles and Responsibilities for Core Team Members of Hospice and Palliative Care Based on Domain of Care

Domain of Care	Disciplines Involved	Role
Physical	Physician/advance practice nurse	Establish care plan with other team members to manage physical symptoms (e.g., pain, shortness of breath, functional decline)
	Nurse	Monitor treatment adherence and effects; identify barriers to treatment plan; coordinate care
	Social worker	Optimize community resources; address psychosocial aspect physical symptoms
	Chaplain	Identify spiritual impacts on physical symptoms and address
Psychological	Physician/advance practice nurse	Ensure mental health support; include access to medications as appropriate
	Nurse	Facilitate mental health support when burden is present; coordinate care plan
	Social worker	Offer and provide counseling, if licensed; recruit necessary community resources
	Chaplain	Identify and engage community spiritual support; provide spiritual support
Spiritual	Physician/advance practice nurse	Report to team spiritual distress, impact on plan of care implementation, and quality of life
	Nurse	Support patient and family; ensure community resources are in place
	Social worker	Recognize spiritual burden and impact on quality of life; offer direct support and/or engage the most appropriate team or community resource as necessary
	Chaplain	Work to address and reduce burden; offer direct spiritual support or connect family with spiritual support; help patient and family identify meaning and work to achieve it
Social	Physician/advance practice nurse	Recognize social burden and its impact on function, nutrition, cognition, and other domains; engage most appropriate team member or community resource
	Nurse	Patient and family support; ensure setting of care matches patient and family goals; coordinate with patient's medical care team
	Social worker	Identify family structure and function and communicate with team to optimize care plans; monitor family's burden from illness
	Chaplain	Optimize community spiritual resources and support family burden

in 2014, the World Health Assembly Resolution on Palliative Care called for all countries to incorporate a palliative care provision into all health care systems (Carrasco et al. 2021).

A substantial barrier to hospice services is that a patient's prognosis must be determined by a physician to be 6 months or less if the illness runs its normal course. This requirement creates unnecessary angst among health care professionals who fear engaging in a direct conversation with a patient to convey that they are dying, uncertainty about the patient's probable course, and fear of referral and hospice rejection of a patient referred too early. Clinicians often struggle when a patient's disease progresses despite optimal medical management and must acknowledge the "failure" of medical intervention to broach a conversation about hospice. Discussion about EoL care is perceived as difficult and time intensive, so too often these conversations are delayed until it is too late. Many patients and families fear that hospice will forgo all treatments except analgesics and anxiolytics, despite the routine use of disease-modifying treatments because they improve symptoms. Patients may also cite financial concerns because they are not aware that hospice services are nearly always reimbursed with little or no out-of-pocket costs.

A barrier to palliative care services outside of the acute care setting relates to the initial focus on symptom management for patients undergoing cancer care. This initial focus resulted in patients with other life-limiting illnesses such as heart, kidney, lung, and neurodegenerative diseases being much less likely to receive palliative and hospice care. Not all hospitals or hospital systems offer palliative care services. Even when available, patients may not be referred due to a lack of service availability, lack of awareness of the resource, or lack of knowledge about when and how to refer. Clinicians may hesitate to refer for fear of upsetting the patient, may see referral as a professional failure, or may not

understand the benefits of referral. Palliative care programs may limit access through overly restrictive eligibility criteria, with such services available only to admitted inpatients. Patients and families may refuse palliative care due to a misunderstanding of the program, may equate palliative care with hospice, or may fear costs and copay requirements.

Taken together, access to palliative care and hospice programs is limited due to several barriers, many of which could be resolved through educational initiatives for health care professionals. Health professionals should be able to accurately identify persons with serious illness, be comfortable talking with patients about their goals of care, and be knowledgeable about the benefits and accessibility of hospice and palliative programs in their communities. Clinicians who can engage in thoughtful conversations about prognosis and disease progression and who can implement shared decision making are ultimately better able to support a patient's care goals.

ADVANCE CARE PLANNING

Advance care planning is a process of engaging a patient in discussion about decisions that might need to be made in the future, considering those decisions ahead of time, and communicating those to both family and health care professionals. These preferences for future care should be documented in the medical record and through specific advance directive documents. Documented wishes go into effect only when the patient is incapacitated and unable to speak for themselves. Advance directives also document patient values and wishes related to EoL care. As a living document, any advance directive should be revisited and can be modified as health, social, or other relevant conditions change.

In addition to advance directives, a patient or their proxy may collaborate with health providers to document physician orders. These documents, such as do not resuscitate orders, are documented in the patient's record. More comprehensive medical orders may be completed as well. In the United States there is some variability in these orders by state. Some examples include the medical orders for scope of treatment (MOLST) or physician orders for life-sustaining treatment (POLST; National POLST, 2022). Individual orders on these forms may differ somewhat by state but generally incorporate decisions about use of cardiopulmonary resuscitation (CPR), artificially administered nutrition and hydration, and medical interventions such as dialysis, ventilation, or blood transfusions. Physician orders documented through advance care planning also include treatment preferences, such as full treatment (e.g., medical and surgical treatments to prolong life or hospital or ICU admission), selected treatments (e.g., restore function such as use of intravenous fluid or positive airway pressure, but not CPR or ICU admission), and/or comfort-focused interventions (e.g., aggressive symptom management while allowing a natural death).

Advance Directives

An advance directive is a document completed by an adult with decision-making capacity (DMC) to help guide decisions about their care in the event they lose the capacity to make health care decisions (see Chapter 3). Patients with DMC maintain the right legally and ethically to accept or refuse any medical treatment. An advance directive helps to extend that right when one loses such capacity. In the United States, the two most commonly used advance directive documents are the durable power of attorney for health care (DPAHC) and living will.

It is a clinician's responsibility to honor a patient's advance directive and to ensure the care plan reflects what has been documented

in the directive. Given that not every scenario can be addressed in an advance directive, what is documented often serves as a general guide on the approach to care for both the care team and the patient's family. In the United States, all states have adopted laws to provide a framework for an advance directive that is generally honored across states (National Conference of Commissioners on Uniform State Laws, 1993). The components within an advance directive should be addressed at least annually or whenever a patient's health substantively changes to ensure the document continues to reflect the patient's current wishes and goals. An advance directive can be changed at any time, with the most recently signed and dated document while capable of decision making being the one that is considered active. If a clinician is unable to honor the patient's clearly stated wishes, then the patient's care should be transferred to a clinician who is willing to follow the directive.

Durable Power of Attorney for Health Care

Adults can designate someone to make decisions on their behalf through a DPAHC document. The named individual is most often called a surrogate decision maker but may also be referred to as a health care proxy, agent, or representative, among other terms (see Table 3–3). A named surrogate speaks for the patient at times when the patient is unable to make decisions for themselves. The surrogate decision maker's responsibility is to decide as the patient would. While most states authorize the surrogate to make decisions to withdraw or withhold life-sustaining treatments, some state statutes limit the authority of a surrogate and set standards of evidence to do so. Most states also have statutes to identify and designate a proxy to act on a patient's behalf when one has not been established. These statutes generally designate the spouse, then adult children, then parents or siblings to act as the patient's surrogate decision maker (see also Chapter 3). The DPAHC form is of particular importance when patients want to name a surrogate decision maker who falls outside the statutory sequence. It is important to note that members of the care team should never serve as a patient's decision maker.

Living Will

Any adult can execute a living will to document individual preferences related to medical intervention in the event that they are dying or permanently unconscious. Living will documents vary by jurisdiction. Often living wills allow an individual to identify only interventions they would *not* want, but in some instances include specifications about desired interventions. Previously documented preferences to forgo (or request) specific interventions can create challenges of interpretation, particularly if documents were completed years earlier than they are applied.

MEDICAL, ETHICAL, AND LEGAL CONSIDERATIONS IN END-OF-LIFE CARE

The alleviation of pain, the optimizing of quality of life, and the provision of comfort as death approaches represent key aims in EoL care. However, fulfilling these objectives is not always straightforward. Physicians, patients, and their families sometimes struggle with challenges in decision making and ethical dilemmas that arise during the process of dying. While working together as a clinical team to reach the best decision for the patient, self-determination is honored through shared decision making to facilitate the process of informed consent (see also Chapter 3). As part of this process, the team helps minimize decision-making burdens so that patients and families can make informed decisions to accept or refuse proposed treatments. This does not require that the clinical team offers all available treatments, particularly options that are not consistent with the standard of care.

Ethical dilemmas develop in the backdrop of uncertainty and most often reveal conflict between competing values. Ethical issues can arise within a family, between a patient and a clinical team, or within a clinical team. For example, as patients lose control of functional abilities or lose meaning in life, these losses may trigger a request for medical assistance in dying (MaiD). Such requests raise ethical and moral questions for patients, family members, and clinicians who must also be familiar with core guiding principles of ethics together with regional legal doctrine. Similarly, patients and families often have to weigh treatment alternatives such as whether to continue burdensome medical treatments with a goal to prolong a person's life or to discontinue medical treatment and allow a natural death. Examples of EoL decisions with ethical and legal implications are provided in Table 1–8.

The core principles of bioethics are considered as part of the decision-making process and include beneficence (promote patient well-being), autonomy (respect for patients' right to self-determination), nonmaleficence (do no harm), and justice (protect vulnerable populations and ensure fair allocation of resources). Ethical considerations require an analysis of fundamental principles of bioethics, which are considered within the patient's unique clinical situation and in conjunction with institutional policies and local, state/provincial, and federal law. It is important to recognize that in a given case, ethical principles may be contradictory to one another and no one principle should be considered more important than another without consideration of the context and all the factors that contribute to each patient's case as unique.

Table 1–8. Ethical and Legal Considerations for Frequently Encountered End-Of-Life Care Issues

End-of-Life Decision	Definition	Ethical/Legal Considerations	Clinical and Other Considerations	Clinical Needs Associated With the Decision
Use of artificially administered nutrition and hydration	Decision to forgo (not start) or withdraw (stop) tube feeding or IV hydration	• Legally and ethically artificially administered food and fluid is a medical treatment that a patient can decline or can stop • Starting and stopping medical intervention (withdrawing) is ethically and legally equivalent to not starting the intervention (withholding)	• Allows patient to die naturally • Discontinues (or does not start) intervention that does not benefit the patient and/or that may cause harm • Evidence-based outcomes data show limited benefit and/or potential harm with use of feeding tubes for patients very near the end of life • Use should be limited to clearly defined therapeutic goal (e.g., tube feeding may benefit patients with head and neck cancer, gastrointestinal cancers with high bowel obstruction, or amyotrophic lateral sclerosis early in the course of the disease) • Counsel patient and family perceptions of "starvation" or dehydration and of food and water as a basic need	• Protocols for comfort feeding, careful handfeeding, and use of ice chips to manage dry mouth contribute to patients' comfort and quality of life • Patient and family education about natural process of dying with expected reduced intake of food and water in the final stages of dying

continues

Table 1–8. *continued*

End-of-Life Decision	Definition	Ethical/Legal Considerations	Clinical and Other Considerations	Clinical Needs Associated With the Decision
Voluntary cessation of eating and drinking	Conscious and deliberate decision by a patient with decision-making capacity and in the end stage of disease to stop accepting food or fluids by mouth, with the purpose of hastening death	A patient has the ethical and legal right to refuse food and fluids at the end of life	Sometimes proposed by patients or families as an alternative to medical assistance in dying	• Patient and family education about natural process of dying with expected reduced intake of food and water in the final stages of dying • Offer comfort feeding as desired, excellent oral care, and oral hydration for comfort
Discontinuation of life sustaining treatment(s)	Decision to stop an intervention that is prolonging the dying process (e.g., ventilator, dialysis, or defibrillator)	• Legally and ethically, medical interventions can be stopped • Starting and stopping medical intervention (withdrawing) is ethically and legally equivalent to not starting the intervention (withholding)	• Patients and families may express a wish to die "without machines" • Allows patient to die naturally	Patient and family education about what to expect, including uncertainties, when the intervention is stopped
Palliative sedation	Lowering patient consciousness using medications to limit patient awareness of pain or suffering that is intractable and intolerable	• Legally permissible practice • Informed consent required and do not resuscitate orders usually accompany	Ethical questions remain about whether or not sedation is appropriate for existential distress	• Must continue treatment for other symptoms such as pain • Patient and family education about what to expect, including uncertainties, associated with sedation

End-of-Life Decision	Definition	Ethical/Legal Considerations	Clinical and Other Considerations	Clinical Needs Associated With the Decision
Physician-assisted death/medical assistance in dying	A physician or other authorized medical practitioner assesses patient and provides, at the patient's request, a combination of lethal medications that the patient can take by their own hand when the patient judges their suffering to be intolerable	• Variability in law by jurisdiction (e.g., legal in Canada, Australia, Belgium, Netherlands, and some U.S. states) • Most laws require verification of terminal condition, limited life expectancy, psychologic assessment, and may require a waiting period	• Should not be equated with decisions to not start (withhold) or stop (withdraw) medical interventions • Remains a controversial practice, but with increasing availability worldwide	• Patient and family education about the process of dying, address fears and concerns including loss of autonomy • Patient education about what to expect, including uncertainties, associated with medical aid in dying
Euthanasia	Voluntary euthanasia: Lethal dose of medication administered with the intent to end the patient's life at the request of a patient Involuntary euthanasia: Lethal dose of medication administered with the intent to end the patient's life with a decision made by someone other than the patient	• Voluntary euthanasia is not permitted in the United States, but is permitted by law in some countries with legal safeguards (e.g., Canada) • Involuntary euthanasia is an illegal in most jurisdictions worldwide	Should not be equated with decisions to not start (withhold) or stop (withdraw) medical interventions or medical aid in dying	Patient and family education about terminology, intent, and alternative options

Comprehensive coverage of bioethics and related legal considerations are beyond the scope of this book. In the face of complex ethical issues, clinicians should access one or more resources to assist in analysis and considerations and to facilitate thoughtful resolution. Most medical centers or systems in the United States, United Kingdom, Canada, and elsewhere have mechanisms for resolution of ethical dilemmas that arise in clinical care through ethics consultation or an ethics committee review (Slowther, 2000). Physicians and nurses with specialty training in hospice and palliative medicine are often well equipped to navigate ethical and legal considerations. The literature abounds with relevant resources and a variety of frameworks to assist clinicians in the careful thought processes needed to resolve complex clinical medical questions (Macauley, 2018).

REFERENCES

Aldridge, M. D., Moreno, J., McKendrick, K., Li, L., Brody, A., & May, P. (2022). Association between hospice enrollment and total health care costs for insurers and families, 2002–2018. *JAMA Health Forum, 3*(2), e215104. https://doi.org/10.1001/jamahealthforum.2021.5104

Back, A., Arnold, B., & Tulsky, J. (2009). *Mastering communication with seriously ill patients: Balancing honesty with empathy and hope.* Cambridge.

Baile, W. F., Buckman, R., Lenzi, R., Glober, G., Beale, E. A., & Kudelka, A. P. (2000). SPIKES —A six-step protocol for delivering bad news: Application to the patient with cancer. *Oncologist, 5*(1), 302–311. https://doi.org/10.1634/theoncologist.5-4-302

Balen, R., Gordon, A. L., Schols, J., Drewes, Y. M., & Achterberg, W. P. (2019). What is geriatric rehabilitation and how should it be organized? A Delphi study aimed at reaching European consensus. *European Geriatric Medicine, 10*(6), 977–987. https://doi.org/10.1007/s41999-019-00244-7

Bumb, M., Keefe, J., Miller, L., & Overcash, J. (2017). Breaking bad news: An evidence-based review of communication models for oncology nurses. *Clinical Journal of Oncology Nursing, 21*(5), 573–580. https://doi.org/10.1188/17.CJON.573-580

Carrasco, J. M., Inbadas, H., Whitelaw, A., & Clark, D. (2021). Early impact of the 2014 World Health Assembly Resolution on Palliative Care: A qualitative study using semistructured interviews with key experts. *Journal of Palliative Medicine, 24*(1), 103–106. https://doi.org/10.1089/jpm.2019.0384

Centers for Medicare and Medicaid Services. (2021). *Medicare benefit policy manual. Chapter 9—Coverage of hospice services under hospital insurance.* https://www.cms.gov/Regulations-and-Guidance/Guidance/Manuals/Downloads/bp102c09.pdf

Childers, J. W., Back, A. L., Tulsky, J. A., & Arnold, R. M. (2017). REMAP: A framework for goals of care conversations. *Journal of Oncology Practice, 13*(10), e844–e850. https://doi.org/10.1200/JOP.2016.018796

Dahl, T. H. (2002). International classification of functioning, disability, and health: An introduction and discussion of its potential impact on rehabilitation services and research. *Journal of Rehabilitation Medicine, 34*(5), 201–204. https://doi.org/10.1080/165019702760279170

Greenstein, J. E., Policzer, J. S., & Shaban, E. S. (2019). Hospice for the primary care physician. *Primary Care, 46*(3), 303–317. https://doi.org/10.1016/j.pop.2019.04.002

Kelley, A. S., & Bollens-Lund, E. (2018). Identifying the population with serious illness: The "denominator" challenge. *Journal of Palliative Medicine, 1*(21 Suppl. 2), S7–S16. https://doi.org/10.1089/jpm.2017.0548

Kelley, A. S., Deb, P., Du, Q., Aldridge Carlson, M. D., & Morrison, R. S. (2013). Hospice enrollment saves money for Medicare and improves care quality across a number of different lengths-of-stay. *Health Affairs (Milwood), 32*(3), 552–561. https://doi.org/10.1377/hlthaff.2012.0851

Khandelwal, N., Curtis, R. J., Freedman, V. A., Kasper, J. D., Gozalo, P., Engelberg, R. A., &

Teno, J. M. (2017). How often is end-of-life care in the United States inconsistent with patients' goals of care? *Journal of Palliative Medicine, 20*(12), 1400–1404. https://doi.org/10.1089/jpm.2017.0065

Kleinpell, R., Vasilevskis, E. E., Fogg, L., & Ely, E. W. (2019). Exploring the association of hospice care on patient experience and outcomes of care. *BMJ Supportive & Palliative Care, 9*(1), e13. https://doi.org/10.1136/bmjspcare-2015-001001

Kyeremanteng, K., Gagnon, L.-P., Thavorn, K., Heyland, D., & D'Egidio, G. (2018). The impact of palliative care consultation in the ICU on length of stay: A systematic review and cost evaluation. *Journal of Intensive Care Medicine, 33*(6), 346–353. https://doi.org/10.1177/0885066616664329

Lunney, J. R., Lynn, J., Foley, D. J., Lipson, S., & Guralnik, J. M. (2003). Patterns of functional decline at the end of life. *Journal of the American Medical Association, 289*(18), 2387–2392. https://doi.org/10.1001/jama.289.18.2387

Lunney, J. R., Lynn, J., & Hogan, C. (2002). Profiles of older Medicare decedents. *Journal of the American Geriatrics Society, 50*(6), 1108–1112. https://doi.org/10.1046/J.1532-5415.2002.50268.X

Macauley, R. C. (2018). *Ethics in palliative care: A complete guide.* Oxford University Press.

Meier, E. A., Gallegos, J. V., Montross-Thomas, L. P., Depp, C. A., Irwin, S. A., & Jeste, D. V. (2016). Defining a good death (successful dying): Literature review and a call for research and public dialogue. *American Journal of Geriatric Psychiatry, 24*(4), 261–271. https://doi.org/10.1016/j.jagp.2016.01.135

Morrison, R. S., & Meier, D. E. (2019). America's care of serious illness: A state-by-state report card on access to palliative care in our nation's hospitals. *Journal of Palliative Medicine, 14*(10), 1094–1096.

National Conference of Commissioners on Uniform State Laws. (1993). *Uniform health-care decisions act.* Uniform Law Commission. https://www.uniformlaws.org/viewdocument/uniform-health-care-decisions-act

National Hospice and Palliative Care Organization. (2021). *Hospice facts and figures.* NHPCO. https://www.nhpco.org/wp-content/uploads/NHPCO-Facts-Figures-2021.pdf

National POLST. (2022). *Honoring the wishes of those with serious illness and frailty.* https://polst.org/

Pollak, K. I., Gao, X., Beliveau, J., Griffith, B., Kennedy, D., & Casarett, D. (2019). Pilot study to improve goals of care conversations among hospitalists. *Journal of Pain & Symptom Management, 58*(5), 864–870. https://doi.org/10.1016/j.jpainsymman.2019.06.007

Robison, J. M., Wilkie, D. J., & Campbell, B. (1995). Sublingual and oral morphine administration. Review and new findings. *The Nursing Clinics of North America, 30*(4), 725–743.

Slowther, A.-M. (2000). Clinical ethics committees. *British Medical Journal, 312*(7262), 649–650. https://doi.org/10.1136/bmj.321.7262.649

Teno, J. M., Clarridge, B. R., Casey, V., Welch, L. C., Wetle, T., Shield, R., & Mor, V. (2004). Family perspectives on end-of-life care at the last place of care. *Journal of the American Medical Association, 291*(1), 88–93.

Wang, C. H., Charlton, B., & Kohlwes, J. (2016). The horrible taste of nectar and honey—Inappropriate use of thickened liquids in dementia: A teachable moment. *JAMA Internal Medicine, 176*(6), 735–736. https://doi.org/10.1001/jamainternmed.2016.1384

Wright, A. A., Zhang, B., Ray, A., Mack, J. W., Trice, E., Balboni, T., . . . Prigerson, H. G. (2008). Associations between end-of-life discussions, patient mental health, medical care near death, and caregiver bereavement adjustment. *Journal of the American Medical Association, 300*(14), 1665–1673. https://doi.org/10.1001/jama.300.14.1665

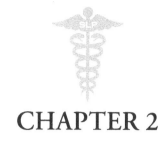

CHAPTER 2

The Roles and Responsibilities of Speech-Language Pathologists in End-of-Life Care

Amanda Stead, Helen Sharp, and Robin Pollens

> *"You matter because you are you, and you matter to the end of your life. We will do all we can, not only to help you die peacefully but also to live until you die."*—Cicely Saunders in Saunders & Clark, 2006

INTRODUCTION

Communication, cognition, eating, drinking, and swallowing are essential for patients as they near the end of life (EoL), and speech-language pathologists (SLPs) have essential knowledge and skills to contribute to the care of patients with life-limiting conditions. SLPs are well prepared to promote patients' ability to communicate directly with their medical team, family, and other loved ones throughout the dying process. SLPs have the knowledge and skills to circumvent barriers to communication, promote safe and comfortable oral feeding, and offer empathy and support to patients, caregivers, and family members.

SLPs serve patients with life-limiting conditions across many settings, including outpatient clinics, inpatient services, home health, long-term care, skilled nursing facilities, and intensive care. No setting is immune from the possibility of patients dying while in the care of an SLP. While this book is centered on patients with known life-limiting conditions, the capacity to provide patient-centered assessment and intervention focused on quality of life for patients who may not recover from their condition has broad application to the work SLPs do in every setting.

Although SLPs possess the necessary skills to serve patients nearing the EoL, clinicians often need clarification about their role in caring for the dying (Chahda et al.,

2017; Collins, 2022). Few training programs in speech-language pathology include coursework or clinical experience in EoL care (Stead et al., 2020; Stead et al., 2023). From a social standpoint, in Westernized countries, discussions about death and dying are rare (Gawande, 2014; Mannix, 2018). Even in clinical contexts, we too often actively avoid confronting the realities of mortality and use countless euphemisms to avoid saying "dead" (Pound, 1936).

When first presented with a referral for a dying patient, clinicians may fear saying the wrong thing or be at a loss for what to say (Mannix, 2018). However, as professionals engage in this work, they report immense satisfaction and even joy (Kirkland, 2017; Mannix, 2018; Twycross, 1997). It is a privilege to help a patient to convey how and where they want to die, or to communicate their goals, fears, symptoms, or final wishes. There is fulfillment when a patient is able to eat a favorite food, when a family member can prepare a favorite dish to nurture their loved one, or when a patient is visibly more comfortable after oral care. It is an honor to provide the tools for a patient to say a final goodbye. The impact of this work holds deep and lasting meaning for family members and the clinicians who serve them.

Clinically, nearly all people who die from progressive diseases experience difficulty with communication, eating, and drinking toward the end of their lives due to systemic weakness and fatigue (Bogaardt et al., 2015). Thus, SLPs should expect referrals for services at any age and in any setting. Ideally, a timely referral for speech-language pathology consultation should be initiated early in the course of illness or disease to allow patients and families access to communication-focused support throughout the course of their disease. In addition, patients near the EoL should be referred for speech-language pathology services when their ability to communicate is a barrier to symptom identification or management or participation in medical decisions or care planning, or if it limits access to social, emotional, or spiritual support (Pollens et al., 2021).

While SLPs often counsel and care for patients at various stages of disease progression across conditions such as head and neck cancer and dementia, unfortunately speech-language pathology services are less frequently sought as the patient gets closer to the end stage of their disease. Appropriate referrals are restricted by medical professionals, patients, and families who are often unfamiliar with the breadth of services SLPs provide and may not recognize the capacity of SLPs to optimize communication and/or functional eating and drinking (O'Reilly & Walshe, 2015). Within the profession of speech-language pathology, the impact of underreferral coupled with little or no explicit training leads to uncertainty about roles and responsibilities. Together these barriers reveal a substantial gap in services that, if filled, would assist members of the care team in providing optimal patient-centered care and enhance the experience of patients and their families. SLPs can and should serve patients and their caregivers throughout the progression toward death, which may extend for weeks, months, or years.

This chapter will highlight the general roles and responsibilities of SLPs in working with adults and children with life-limiting conditions. We will address service delivery models in this chapter and expand on the role of the SLP through direct service to patients, indirect service, and consultation. Barriers to services and ways to overcome those barriers are addressed together with special considerations for SLPs, such as the relationship between speech-language pathology services and spiritual care for patients nearing the EoL. Finally, we address goal writing, and the chapters that follow provide a more specific focus on assessment and treatment for adults with communication and cognition needs (Chapter 4), adults with dysphagia (Chapter 5), and the role of the SLP in working with children with life-limiting conditions (Chapter 6).

WHAT PATIENTS NEED TO COMMUNICATE AS THEY NEAR THE END OF LIFE

When people are told or become aware that they have limited time left to live, their priorities and interests may shift in a variety of ways, including a focus on comfort and basic needs, a desire to reach closure in relationships, a need to confront spiritual and existential questions of meaning, and more (Egan,

2017). Communication is essential to achieve individualized end-of-life goals and to meet essential physical, social, psychological, and emotional needs.

ROLES AND RESPONSIBILITIES OF THE SPEECH-LANGUAGE PATHOLOGIST IN END-OF-LIFE CARE

Speech-language services for individuals with life-limiting conditions are in the scope of practice and well-defined as best practice (American Academy of Hospice and Palliative Medicine, n.d; American Speech-Language-

---

What Do Patients Need to Communicate as They Near the End of Life?

- Report physiologic changes
  - describe symptoms including dizziness, pain, nausea, constipation, fatigue
- Understand information from care providers
  - receive information about medical tests and care plan options
- Request basic care needs
  - pain management
  - toileting needs
  - positioning (within the bed, move to chair)
  - general comfort (too warm, too cold)
  - hunger, thirst, and preferences for specific foods
- Engage in meaningful discussions about their care
  - develop a plan of care with the medical team

- complete advance directives (living will, durable power of attorney for health care)
- complete advance care wishes and medical orders (e.g., POLST form)
- Engage in meaningful conversations with others
  - discuss wishes with family and friends
  - share memories with family, friends, colleagues
  - obtain spiritual guidance
- Plan for the end of life or after death
  - put legal and financial affairs in order
  - provide instructions for funeral or celebration of life plans
  - contribute to obituary

Hearing Association, n.d.; Centers for Medicare and Medicaid Services, 2021). In addition, the literature in communication sciences and disorders provides further details about the scope and role of SLPs (Bogaardt et al., 2015; Brownlee & Bruening, 2012; Chahda et al., 2017; Pollens, 2004, 2012, 2020; Pollens & Lynn, 2011; Schleinich et al., 2008; Sharp & Payne, 1998; Stead & McDonnell, 2015; Toner & Shadden, 2012; Wallace, 2013).

> *"…there is, indisputably, a role for SLPs in the field of adult palliative care, particularly in the domains of communication and swallowing."*—Chahda and colleagues, 2017, p. 67

Speech-Language Services Recognized by Professional Organizations and Payors

Communication is essential to patient-centered palliative care (Dunne, 2005). Professional standards of care recognize speech-language services as a requirement for high-quality hospice and palliative care services. These standards of care are also reflected in reimbursement guidelines.

Professional Organizations and Standards of Care

The American Speech-Language-Hearing Association (ASHA), the American Academy of Hospice and Palliative Medicine (AAHPM), and the National Consensus Project for Quality Palliative Care (2018) all identify an essential role for SLPs in hospice and palliative care. ASHA identifies that speech-language pathology services contribute "to the overall quality of life of patients nearing the end of life" and describes the role of intervention as

"not rehabilitative, but facilitative" (ASHA, n.d.). AAHPM and the Accreditation Council for Graduate Medical Education (ACGME) identify SLPs as interdisciplinary team members for hospice and palliative care teams. It is expected that board-certified physicians are familiar with the roles and responsibilities of SLPs and refer to SLPs to meet patient goals and needs.

Medicare Guidelines

Medicare recognizes and reimburses services for hospice services and requires an interdisciplinary team model of care. Medicare covers speech-language pathology services under the hospice benefit "for purposes of symptom control or to enable the individual to maintain activities of daily living and basic functional skills" (Centers for Medicare and Medicaid Services, 2021, §40.1.8). Medicare requires that speech-language pathology services be available as a condition of participation in hospice and palliative care programs (§418.72). It is essential for SLPs in the United States to be familiar with Medicare guidelines, even when working with patients who do not receive Medicare because most hospitals and insurance companies in the United States view Medicare guidelines as a standard for coverage and care requirements.

International Guidelines

The World Health Organization (WHO, 2016) includes communication as an essential component of palliative care practice that allows patients to engage in their care plan and effective pain and symptom management. Speech-language pathology services are identified as part of hospice and/or palliative care in most countries in which speech-language pathology is a recognized profession. Guidelines for hospice and palliative care services include SLPs across many countries (e.g.,

Health Canada, 2018; Hong Kong Institute of Speech Therapists, 2021; Royal College of Speech and Language Therapists, 2023).

Medical Literature

The role of the SLP as a provider of communication, cognition, and swallowing assessment and intervention is described in the medical literature. Roles for the SLP include (a) consultation with patients, families, and members of the hospice team in the areas of communication, cognition, and swallowing; (b) direct and indirect strategies to support communication and the patient's role in decision making, to maintain social relationships, and to fulfill EoL goals; (c) direct and indirect strategies to optimize eating, drinking, and swallowing function to improve comfort and satisfaction and maintenance of social roles; and (d) as a member of to the interdisciplinary care team (Chahda et al., 2017; Pollens, 2004). SLPs may also consider ethical and legal factors; offer support related to the communication of patients' emotional, existential, and spiritual concerns; and/or participate in EoL care research (Chahda et al., 2017).

SLP KNOWLEDGE AND SKILLS APPLY TO END-OF-LIFE CARE

SLPs support patients with life-limiting conditions in ways that may differ from the traditional focus of rehabilitation. However, the knowledge and skills SLPs employ across settings also apply to assessing and supporting adults and children with life-limiting conditions. SLPs bring deep knowledge of barriers to communication, cognition, eating, and drinking and a host of ways in which these barriers can be circumvented. Although the outcome for the patient is death, the focus of palliative and EoL care is to maximize the

patient's capacity while alive. Any outcome that makes communication, eating, or drinking easier is a success. Any outcome that allays the fears or builds the confidence of a caregiver is a success. Any outcome that supports the patient's preference(s) for care is a success. The SLP's expertise can also facilitate the work of other care team members, thereby improving the overall quality of care for the patient and their family.

Patient-Centered Assessment and Treatment Approaches

Patient-centered assessment and treatment are central to every aspect of patient care, and this philosophy is exemplified in the context of imminent decline or death. In this context, SLPs may only see a patient for a single consultation or may follow a patient over weeks, months, or even years.

Before initiating the assessment, the SLP should establish patient and caregiver goals and preferences. At the outset, the SLP should assess the patient's understanding of their situation. Clinicians can use questions such as "What can you tell me about your condition?" and "What changes have you noticed recently?" to identify the patient's awareness and/or willingness to discuss their clinical status and trajectory. For more discussion about communication to establish patients' preferences, see Chapters 1 and 3.

Standardized assessments are rarely of value in this context. Instead, the SLP should conduct a meaningful informal assessment with a focus on how best to meet the patient's goals (Chahda et al., 2017). Some examples of intervention strategies will be addressed in this chapter, and specific strategies and example goals are available related to adult communication and cognition (Chapter 4), dysphagia (Chapter 5), and pediatric populations (Chapter 6).

Counseling and Communication Skills Essential for End-of-Life Conversations

Excellent counseling and communication skills often allow SLPs to establish rapport quickly. The relationship between clinician and patient is most effective when individuals can form a therapeutic alliance (Eubanks et al., 2018), which is enhanced through a focus on the patient's primary goals. In addition, effective counseling techniques can solidify the clinician–patient relationship and offer the patient and family meaningful psychosocial support. See Table 2–1 for examples of effective counseling techniques when working with a patient near the EoL.

Determining Patient Preferences

Patient self-determination is highly valued in hospice and palliative care services. For patients and families to make decisions that align with their goals and values, they must understand their circumstances and the options available and have time to make informed decisions. Unfortunately, medical information is often complex, laden with jargon, and overwhelming, particularly in the context of new or complex changes in health status. More detailed discussion about the components of informed consent is provided in Chapter 3.

The SLP may be a suitable partner to support physicians, nurses, social workers, and other professionals in communication of medical information and difficult discussions around care plans. SLPs can serve patients and families by optimizing the delivery of complex information and ensuring the patient and family understand the nature of the patient's condition and available options. Patients and their families often need time to process new information about their condition, consider the options available, ask questions, and come

to terms with death. Information may need to be repeated or provided through multiple modalities to ensure excellent comprehension, even in the absence of a communication disorder.

The role of the SLP is even more essential when patients have a communication disorder. When there are barriers to the patient or caregiver's comprehension, the SLP can assist the medical care team in optimizing information delivery based on the patient's language and cognitive skills. For example, a patient with aphasia may be able to understand when information is broken into small chunks or provided in multiple modalities. Similarly, for patients with limited speech or language expression, the SLP may be able to provide tools or strategies to increase the patient's intelligibility or language expression.

Truth Telling and Breaking Bad News

One essential aspect of building trust is honesty. Although on the surface, truth telling is an intuitive and worthy goal, in practice, clinicians experience uncertainty about how and when to implement truth telling in clinical contexts. It can be daunting for a clinician to deliver bad news or say "I don't know" when a patient or family asks a difficult question. However, clinicians who embody humility and grace build trust with patients even in uncertainty.

In the context of EoL care, clinicians are frequently faced with communicating complex and difficult-to-hear information. Clinicians experience personal stress and discomfort about being the messenger of bad news (Fallowfield & Jenkins, 2004) and concurrently fear they will cause distress (Fallowfield & Jenkins, 2004; Mannix, 2018). Little has been written about breaking bad news in speech-language pathology, and few programs teach students how to break bad news. Nevertheless, SLPs frequently present a new diagnosis,

Table 2–1. Description and Examples of Counseling Techniques Useful in End-of-Life Care

Counseling Technique	Description	Examples
Validation	Validation within therapy *encourages and supports* the understanding and acceptance of the client's experiences, both verbally and nonverbally. It signifies that clients are heard and that their behavior is understandable (even if not appropriate) in their given context.	"It must have felt difficult to open up about that. Thank you for sharing!" "Yeah, I can see how that might make you feel really sad." "It makes sense you would be so upset about that." "I'm here." "I can see that you are very (upset, sad, frightened, scared . . .)" "I'm so sorry you are experiencing this. I am here to support you."
Verbal following	Verbal following combines listening and repeating verbatim. Listen carefully to what the client says and then repeat back a few words of the message. This strategy aids health care professionals (HCPs) in (a) paying attention and following the content of the client's message; (b) showing respect for the client's ideas, feelings, and language of expression; and (c) encouraging the client to keep talking.	Client says: "But what is going to happen when people can't understand me as well? I don't want people talking about me like I'm not even there." Clinician response: "You don't want people to talk about you like you aren't even there." Client says: "Right because then it will feel like I'm not a part of my own life. I want to be able to talk to my family."
Paraphrasing and reflection	Paraphrasing is a form of responding empathically to the emotions of another person by repeating in other words what this person said while focusing on the essence of what they feel and what is important to them.	Client says: "It just isn't fair that this is happening right now. I was hoping to be able to make it to my granddaughter's wedding in the fall but it seems like that isn't going to happen. I'm not even sure they're going to be able to visit me since they live so far away." Clinician says: "It sounds like you are really disappointed that you may not get to see your granddaughter again."
Open-ended questions	Open-ended questions provide the client with maximum latitude on where to begin talking and what to say. They are nondirective strategies because the clinician makes no assumptions about what topic to choose or in what direction the conversation should go.	"What's on your mind?" "What makes you say that?" "What are you hoping for?" "What is something you are hoping to achieve through our work together?"

discuss the implications of a diagnosis, confirm a diagnosis, or discuss clinical findings with patients and families (Gold & Gold, 2018; Sterling et al., 2013).

Strategies for breaking bad news are well described in the medical literature, and skill-focused training programs are available (see Table 1–3 in Chapter 1 for examples). Effective communication of bad news requires preparation and intentional use of strategies. Clinicians should signal that they hold difficult news and ensure available space and time. Before the meeting, clinicians should consider what key points they wish families to take away from the conversation (Fallowfield & Jenkins, 2004; Ngo-Metzger et al., 2008).

Clinicians routinely underestimate the degree to which they use medical jargon when communicating with patients and families (Castro et al., 2007). The use of medical jargon negatively impacts patients' understanding of their condition and disproportionately impacts outcomes for patients with low health literacy (Graham & Brookey, 2008; Rimmer, 2014). In addition to avoiding professional jargon, clinicians should communicate small portions of information at a time and use straightforward vocabulary to name and explain conditions (Pitt & Hendrickson, 2020).

Research has shown that, particularly during emotional conversations, patients retain between 20% and 60% of the medical information provided by clinicians (Kessels, 2003). This means that it is essential that one or two critical points are prioritized and delivered to optimize understanding and support decision making. In addition, clinicians should expect to review and repeat information already given in subsequent appointments.

> *"We rely on euphemism, silence, and jargon when we most acutely need to be clear and articulate."*—Puri, 2019

All interactions with patients and families should consider the individual's preferences and lived experiences (Fallowfield & Jenkins, 2004; Girgis & Sanson-Fisher, 1998; Ngo-Metzger et al., 2008). SLPs can provide empathy and support during difficult conversations using language grounded in counseling techniques (Holland & Nelson, 2018; Luterman, 2016). Thoughtful and caring delivery of news, coupled with empathetic responses that acknowledge and validate the patient's emotions, creates an environment of trust that can be built on to support an honest discussion of options and shared decision making (Fallowfield & Jenkins, 2004; Manderson & Warren, 2010).

> **Case Study: Breaking Bad News**
>
> The SLP checks on a patient with advanced dementia. The patient's daughter is attempting to feed her mother and tearfully asks for help. The SLP recognizes that this is an opportunity to explore if the patient's daughter understands that her mother's interest in food will decline as her dementia advances. The SLP considers that the daughter may benefit from the reassurance that her mother's poor intake is a characteristic of the disease, not a failure of her care and skill. The SLP also recognizes that this discussion heightens awareness of the patient's decline and prepares for an emotional response from the patient's daughter and the possibility of entering a discussion about goals of care related to eating, drinking, and swallowing.

Table 1–3 in Chapter 1 details examples of available training programs and standardized approaches to goals of care conversations.

For example, the REMAP program (Childers et al., 2017) is a framework to support clinicians in seeking understanding and remaining flexible during difficult conversations. Initiating a conversation with a "headline" lets the patient or family know things are in a different place. In the case example, the clinician might use the headline, "Your mother's decline in interest in eating is a normal part of the disease. It is not a reflection of your skill in feeding her."

Familiarity With the Medical and Physiologic Aspects of Dying

The knowledge and skills required for SLPs to serve patients nearing the EoL are no different from the knowledge and skills required across settings. As is the case in any area of practice, there are additional areas of knowledge that contribute to the SLP's ability to offer appropriate, evidence-based care. These include awareness of the physiologic stages of dying, which are summarized in Chapter 1. Clinicians who work with palliative care or hospice teams should develop further knowledge of the dying process. However, even with a deep understanding of the trajectory of physiologic changes that lead to death, clinical predictions about precisely when a patient will die are notoriously inaccurate. Nonetheless, clinicians should learn and recognize predictable changes in cognition, physical stamina, and physiologic status that occur in the weeks and days before death. For example, the SLP should be aware that decreased oral intake and weight loss are expected and be prepared to offer assurance to caregivers who may feel responsible or inadequate as they observe these changes in the patient's health. Awareness of the trajectory of dying assists the SLP in communicating with the care team and discussing care goals with the patient and family. For SLPs who work with patients with degenera-tive diseases, attention to the patient's overall health status is relevant because the SLP may be among the first professionals to note a decline in a patient's function that signals readiness for palliative or hospice care (Pollens, 2012; Roe & Leslie, 2010).

SLPs working in palliative or hospice care services should understand the impact of physiologic changes in degenerative disease and how these changes impact communication and swallowing as patients' function declines. For example, weight loss alters the way dentures fit, negatively impacting chewing, swallowing, and speech intelligibility. As the SLP assesses oral function for speech and swallowing, careful attention to oral health is also highly relevant for children and adults as they near the EoL (Krikheli et al., 2018). Dry mouth, cracked lips, oral thrush (Candidiasis), dental pain, ill-fitting dentures, and poor oral hygiene are common symptoms that patients and caregivers often disregard near the EoL (Gustafsson et al., 2021; Magnani et al., 2019). SLPs are well aware that good oral hygiene reduces the risk of pneumonia from oral sources of infection, including in patients who are tube fed (Maeda & Akagi, 2014). It is also well documented that oral care is essential to patient comfort (McCann et al., 1994; Schofield et al., 2022; Venkatasalu et al., 2020). Thus, by ensuring that these symptoms are addressed, the SLP can contribute to the patient's comfort and well-being in the end-stages of life.

In conjunction with understanding patterns of physiological decline and frequently observed impact on speech, language, cognitive and oral intake, and swallow function, SLPs should develop basic knowledge of the medications most frequently used in EoL care and common side effects. Table 2–2 summarizes medications that impact cognition. Pain medication is frequently used to meet the goal of symptom management in palliative and hospice medicine. Among the most

Table 2–2. Examples of Prescription Medications That Can Cause Cognitive Impairment

Mechanism of Cognitive Impairment	Classes of Medications
Sedation	Antihistamines, anticholinergics, benzodiazepines, antipsychotics, nonbenzodiazepine sedative hypnotics, barbiturates, urinary incontinence agents, antidepressants, analgesics
Confusion	Antihistamines, urinary incontinence agents, antipsychotics, cardiovascular agents, analgesics
Amnesia	Benzodiazepines, gastrointestinal agents
Delirium	Anticholinergics, opioid analgesics, benzodiazepine and nonbenzodiazepine sedative hypnotics

Source: From *Medical setting considerations for the speech-language pathologist* (pp. 1–154) by Spencer, K. A., & Daniels, J. Copyright © 2020 Plural Publishing, Inc. All rights reserved. Used with permission.

commonly used medications for pain control is morphine, with known side effects including dry mouth, sedation, mild myoclonus (muscle twitch), and constipation (Glare et al., 2016). The risks and management of constipation are not often discussed in the training of SLPs. However, SLPs should understand that the impact of constipation can include nausea, vomiting, and lack of appetite, which can then be mistakenly connected with disinterest in food and difficulty with feeding, eating, or swallowing.

Similarly, it is rare for SLPs to receive direct training in pharmacology, but because so many medications can impact cognition, speech, eating, and swallowing, SLPs who work with patients with life-limiting conditions should be acquainted with medication classes and side effects. They should inquire about medications as part of each assessment and at the start of each intervention session. Frequently used classes of medications and their side effects are summarized in Chapter 1 (see also Table 1–5). For example, suppose a patient with chronic pain managed with opioids is referred for evaluation. In that case, the SLP will likely maximize the value of an assessment if the patient is seen within an hour after taking pain medications. Optimally, the patient will be comfortable and able to participate but not overly drowsy.

Familiarity With Bioethics and Legal Distinctions

All care team members must have an excellent understanding of the terminology of hospice, palliative care, and bioethics to avoid contributing to or exacerbating misunderstandings. For example, caregivers often misconstrue discussing forgoing tube feeding as "euthanasia" or direct "killing" of the patient, which is not the case. If the SLP is familiar with the terminology of bioethics as it relates to the artificial administration of food and fluids they can support patients and families as they express their preferences for intake of food and/or fluid. SLPs who work in the context of palliative or hospice care should build knowledge of the core terminology of hospice, palliative care, and EoL care as part of the interprofessional team. Core terminology is introduced in Chapters 1 and 3.

SPECIAL CONSIDERATIONS BY SETTING

The primary responsibilities of assessment, intervention, and patient–caregiver education and counseling are consistent across settings. However, there are some variations and special considerations for the delivery of EoL care by setting.

Acute Care or Intensive Care

Inpatient acute care, critical care, or intensive care is an overwhelming setting for patients and their families. The environment is noisy, filled with intimidating equipment and a dizzying array of professionals who each have a role in keeping the patient stable and alive. In this context, the goals and strategies of care can change quickly. Whether the patient is admitted with a catastrophic change in health status due to injury, new onset health problem, or rapid decline or exacerbation of a chronic condition, patients and their families can be expected to be ill prepared for this environment and to confront unexpected end-of-life decisions.

When patients require intensive care, they are often very ill, heavily medicated, and/or orally intubated, thus unable to communicate. If the SLP can establish a means of communication that is of substantial value. In circumstances in which the patient cannot provide direction for their care, families are often asked to make treatment decisions without clear directives or discuss care goals with the patient (see also Chapter 3 for further discussion of advance care planning). The burden of these decisions on family members is substantial.

Research by Levin and colleagues (2010) found that 54% of family members contending with EoL decisions in an intensive care

unit (ICU) lacked a strong understanding of patient diagnosis, treatment plan, or prognosis. Additionally, 40% of family members perceived a conflict with ICU staff, with most reporting unprofessional behavior, such as overheard breaches of confidentiality or insensitive remarks.

Due to the professional care team's knowledge of intensive care, patient health status, and physiologic aspects of dying, it is common for professional care team members to conclude that the patient is dying before the patient's family accepts this status. This gap in knowledge requires that clinicians practice clear communication, empathy, excellent listening, and family-centered communication. In addition, it is essential to recognize that the distress and confusion of the setting mean that otherwise competent adults will demonstrate signs of cognitive overload. So, although the family "has been told," professionals should expect to repeat information, provide time (where able) to make decisions, and offer empathy and support to caregivers in crisis.

Home-Based Hospice or Home Health

Home health SLPs often follow patients with degenerative conditions over a long period. For example, SLPs often provide services for patients with degenerative diseases such as Parkinson's disease, motor neuron disease, dementia, or chronic obstructive pulmonary disease (COPD). In this context, SLPs build strong relationships with patients and caregivers. As a result, SLPs may be among the first to notice a substantive decline in the patient's physical and/or cognitive health status and identify readiness for palliative or hospice care (Pollens, 2012).

In the United States, most hospice services are provided in the patient's home. There are several advantages to home-based care. For patients with many life-limiting conditions, it is easier for them and their caregivers both physically and cognitively to remain at home rather than navigate appointments, travel, parking, and other aspects of outpatient clinic visits. A home environment reduces anxiety and loss of control frequently observed in hospital settings. Although patients and families retain more autonomy in their own homes, they remain vulnerable to the power differential between clinician and patient and to a sense of loss of control as the home becomes a center of care. Therefore, clinicians who work in home health or home hospice must embody humility and respect as they enter a patient's home.

Clinicians learn a great deal about a patient's function and needs from direct observation of the patient's home setting and can provide appropriate, individualized recommendations. For example, it is beneficial to see how the patient is positioned in a recliner or bed and be able to provide on-site instruction to family members. Similarly, medications, glasses, hearing aids, augmentative and alternative communication (AAC) devices, and other frequently forgotten items are usually present and accessible in the patient's home. Working in a patient's environment allows the SLP to identify individual needs or activities that can be addressed. These may be simple changes, such as posting a clock, calendar, or whiteboard in the patient's room to assist with orientation and let the patient know what to expect. These environmental supports may be particularly important if the family has set up a hospital bed in a space that was used as a den, or living or dining area. The needs of the home care partners can also be directly observed, which can facilitate the development of authentic goals and interventions. For example, the SLP may note that a patient's family member has difficulty with vocal loudness and recommends using a voice amplifier to reduce the burden on the family member and the patient in conversation together with identification of background noise, such as an unattended television in an adjacent room. Service delivery in the patient's home requires flexibility, creativity, and problem solving. Being with a person in their own home can lead to more open discussion, personal reflection, and accurate identification of needs. The SLP can be an empathic listener and enter into a true partnership with the patient in this context.

Hospice or Palliative Care Centers

Patients admitted to inpatient hospice units or in-residence hospice centers are typically very ill and near the expected death time. However, some patients are admitted for a short stay associated with caregiver respite needs. The SLP may be consulted to offer strategies to support communication for decision making and/or pain and symptom management. In most inpatient hospice services, speech-language pathology assessment and intervention will be limited to one or two visits.

Patients Not Enrolled in Hospice or Palliative Care

Unfortunately, many patients nearing the EoL are not formally managed under a hospice or palliative care designation. Most often, patients who could benefit from a palliative care approach or referral for hospice services are not referred at all or referral occurs very late in their disease trajectory. In other cases, the patient or family may reject a timely referral or enrollment in hospice care despite eligibility.

Without a team-based hospice or palliative care approach, SLPs may be confronted with challenging discussions about goals of care or advance care planning because the patient and family are not fully informed about their medical status or remain in denial about the seriousness of their health status. SLPs with long-standing relationships with patients and families, such as home health, skilled nursing, outpatient services, or other long-term care relationships, may serve as a bridge to palliative and hospice services.

MODELS OF SPEECH-LANGUAGE PATHOLOGY SERVICE DELIVERY

Traditional Rehabilitation-Focused Services Modified for End-of-Life Care

"Traditional" rehabilitation services focus on restoring function lost due to injury or illness. This service delivery model follows a predictable pattern of referral, assessment, intervention, and follow-up, often over a relatively long period. When patients have a terminal illness, rehabilitation-focused services are appropriate when services align with the patient's goals and these may focus on adequate rather than optimal function (Twycross, 1981; Sharp & Payne, 1998). Rehabilitation services offered in conjunction with palliative care have been described across four primary types of service delivery by Javier and Montagnini (2011):

- preventive
- restorative
- supportive
- palliative

Speech-language pathology services viewed within the restricted scope of traditional restorative services have contributed to the unfounded belief that individuals no longer on a restorative trajectory do not benefit from rehabilita-

tive services from allied health professionals, including physical and occupational therapy as speech-language pathology services. Unfortunately, this viewpoint is too often held by medical professionals, patients, families, and rehabilitation professionals themselves. This misguided approach contributes to low referral rates and uncertainty about roles and responsibilities when referrals are received.

In care for individuals with life-limiting conditions, the pathway from referral to assessment, intervention, and follow-up remains the same. However, both timeline and mode of service delivery may differ. In the context of hospice and palliative care referrals, SLPs deliver care through direct assessment or intervention with the patient, indirect services such as training communication partners, or consultation with the primary team of professional care providers. In addition, SLPs may serve as consultants to other palliative team members to support specific case management questions.

Direct Service Delivery

SLPs may work directly with the patient to evaluate their current function, most often conducted using informal assessment techniques to assess comprehension, language expression, speech intelligibility, and cognitive status and/or to identify concerns related to eating, drinking, and swallowing. Based on the assessment of function, the SLP may work directly with the patient to support language comprehension, teach strategies for language production (e.g., word retrieval) and cognition including orientation to place and time, provide and instruct the patient in the use of an AAC device, and/or implement strategies to support safe eating or drinking. Intervention strategies may be introduced in the same session in which the evaluation takes place to meet the patient's immediate needs.

If the SLP follows the patient over time, it is essential to note that variability in performance is expected within and between appointments. In addition, side effects of medication and the patient's health status contribute to short- and medium-term variation in physical and cognitive function.

The SLP should be aware of the patient's status through notes from other health providers and discussion with the patient's primary nurse and/or family members and should include relevant information in the documentation of assessment or intervention. However, direct clinical interactions with patients may be brief or restricted by the volume of health providers, patient and family fatigue, and/or interest in services.

Indirect Service Delivery: Caregiver Education and Training

An essential component of working with patients near the EoL is training their caregivers, family and friends, and professional team members. Caregivers are integral to EoL care in all cases, and indirect services should be blended with direct services. Caregivers are best positioned to implement strategies that increase patient safety and comfort (Chandregowda et al., 2021). Sometimes the patient will be too ill or fatigued to participate in direct service delivery, and the primary focus of the intervention will be caregiver education and training.

A frequent goal of indirect service delivery is to work with the caregiver to optimize communication. For example, the SLP may coach a family member to ask effective yes/no questions and to allow adequate time for the patient to respond (Chandregowda et al., 2021). When caregivers can optimize communication function, the outcome is decreased distress for both patient and family through-

out dying (Garrett et al., 2007). Chandregowda and colleagues (2021) prepared a caregiver handout to provide those caring for someone near the EoL with tangible strategies to maximize interaction with their loved one. These strategies are beneficial and can be modified for use across settings. Suggestions for caregivers include attending to body language, remaining positive, trying to communicate even when they are having difficulty, and minimizing background noise and others (Chandregowda et al., 2021).

Similarly, SLPs can support caregiver knowledge and skills to achieve safer and more effective approaches to eating and drinking and/or to maintain focus on the patient's comfort as they experience physiologic decline. The SLP may encourage family members to prepare small meals and snacks to be consumed throughout the day rather than three larger meals when the patient or family expresses concern about diminished intake during meals. As the patient's health declines, the SLP may reinforce the family's understanding of what to expect and how best to offer care. Caregivers are not necessarily aware that a decline in intake is expected as patients near end-stage disease. It is counterintuitive to many people that pushing the patient to eat and drink increases discomfort (Bogaardt et al., 2015). If caregivers are prepared and know what to expect, some of the stress and negative emotional impact associated with caring for someone near the EoL can be reduced (Williams, 2018). As the patient nears death, caregivers are often uncertain about what to do but want to continue to care for the patient. When the patient is no longer interested in eating or is unable to eat or drink, it is vital to teach caregivers that excellent oral care enhances patient comfort (Magnani et al., 2019; Soileau & Elster, 2018) and train them to provide oral care. Direct teaching raises awareness of the need for oral care and offers a way for family members to provide care for their loved ones (Schofield et al., 2022).

Consultative Model

One of the primary roles that SLPs can serve for patients near the EoL is as a consultant to the medical care team. When an SLP does not serve as a standing member of a hospice or palliative care team, the consultative model is a way for the SLP to communicate with the interdisciplinary team and provide discipline-specific knowledge to support patient care for an individual patient or across the caseload. For example, SLPs may be asked to consult about communication, cognition, feeding, or swallowing. This approach contrasts with the traditional "referral for assessment or therapy" approach. For example, the SLP may train team members who conduct home visits to support functional communication for hearing aid users by teaching the steps for a hearing aid listening check, battery replacement, and hearing aid placement.

The SLP may work with the care team to develop standard approaches to support current and future patients. Broad-based training for the care team to identify speech, language, hearing, cognition, and/or dysphagia concerns, to understand the impact of each of these concerns for patients, and when to refer for speech-language services. Examples of direct, indirect, and consultation approaches and strategies are summarized by the rehabilitation model in Table 2–3.

The SLP could work with specific team members, such as the nurse and social worker, to develop a standard low-tech AAC device to take to all initial intake interviews. In addition, the SLP may contribute screening questions to assist with the identification of communication or swallowing concerns during the intake and/or ongoing medical assessment processes.

Lastly, the SLP may work in consultation with the hospice team to support their work with a given patient. For example, the SLP may guide a nurse to use Supported Conversation techniques (Kagan, 1998) when working with a patient with aphasia.

GOAL WRITING

SLPs who work in the United States and elsewhere often raise questions about whether speech-language pathology and other rehabilitation services are reimbursable when a patient is not expected to show gains in function. Despite stringent guidelines that require evidence of patient progress in some areas of practice, Medicare requires speech-language pathology services to be available as a condition for funding any hospice program (Centers for Medicare and Medicaid Services, 2011).

The SLP's goals in the context of EoL care focus on patient comfort and symptom management. Creating patient-centered goals that align with the overall goals of palliative care has a meaningful impact on the patient and the family. SLPs should also consider the needs and goals of other palliative care team members as they work to maximize the patient's comfort and quality of care. Hospice and palliative care hold the patient's wishes at the center of the care plan, so many of the hospice team's goals are best met through direct communication with the patient. For example, the social worker aims to understand the client's emotional concerns related to dying and their preference for dying at home or in an inpatient setting. A patient's ability to communicate their experience of pain is immensely valuable to achieving the goal of adequate pain control. Therefore, the SLP

Table 2–3. Models of Rehabilitation Applied to SLP Services in End-of-Life Care

Rehabilitation Model		Type of Intervention	Examples
Preventive	Direct	SLP counsels patient about likelihood of decline in speech intelligibility	Facilitate early access and practice with alternative communication device while patient can provide direct input through spoken language
	Indirect	SLP works with patient's spouse to identify core vocabulary list	Spouse provides list of family members' names
	Consultation	Inservice for hospice intake team	Ensure hospice intake process includes note of sensory supports (glasses, hearing aids)
Rehabilitative	Direct	Intervention to optimize function in speech, language, cognitive, or swallowing function	Brief intervention to teach patient to alternate bites of food and sips of liquid to help clear oral cavity
	Indirect	Support family caregivers to enact strategies to maximize patient's swallow function	Teach spouse how to position the patient for meal time
	Consultation	Develop referral criteria for speech-language and cognitive function assessment and intervention with palliative care service	Build infographic for palliative care physicians and nurses to identify when to refer patients for SLP services
Supportive	Direct	Maximize patient capacity to communicate basic needs	Ensure living space has accessible aid to facilitate communication and independence
	Indirect	Train family and other care providers related to speech, language, or dysphagia	Orient primary physician to use short phrases and sentences when communicating plans for a patient with aphasia
	Consultation	Build resources for hospice team to provide families	Create laminated card with sample yes/no questions
Palliative	Direct	Maximize patient capacity to communicate basic needs	Teach patient use of low-tech AAC to request pain medication
	Indirect	Coach family caregivers with evidence-based comfort measures	Train spouse to complete routine oral care and hygiene to replace food preparation and feeding

Table 2–3. *continued*

Rehabilitation Model		Type of Intervention	Examples
Palliative *continued*	Consultation	Build awareness and understanding of patient's level of language comprehension	Encourage family and care team members to talk about the patient with the assumption they understand what is being said about them

Note. In some settings the consultation model is not reimbursable; however, these strategies can be incorporated in the work of the SLP as part of effective interdisciplinary team care.
Sources: Chahda et al. (2017); Pollens (2004, 2012).

should ensure the intervention goals directly serve the patient's current needs. Table 2–4 provides example goals. Please also see goals related to communication and cognition (Chapter 4); goals to support eating, drinking, and swallowing (Chapter 5); and goals for children (Chapter 6).

The care team is more likely to value speech-language pathology services when they can see the direct connection between the outcomes of speech-language pathology services and the achievement goals of care they have established for that patient (Pollens, 2020). For example, a patient can report changes in pain to the nurse and concerns about funeral planning to the social worker using a picture board. These positive outcomes serve to educate the team about the value and relevance of SLP intervention in EoL care.

Barriers and Considerations for Goal Writing

EoL care takes place across many settings, and documentation requirements vary by setting. At times, electronic medical records (EMRs) are utilized, which may require SLPs to write goals using an established template. The template may not align with a palliative or EoL

care framework. Some suggestions for writing EoL care goals within an EMR system:

- Suppose the SLP is required to select a goal from an existing template in the EMR. In that case, they should select the closest reasonable goal and use a dialogue box to clarify the goal or establish a focus of intervention. For example:
  - Best template approximation of the goal: Patient will improve verbal production for conversation with minimal cues at 80% accuracy.
  - Dialogue box note: Communication goal focuses on maintaining social connection and expressing preferences for EoL care.
- If the SLP can edit the template, two new goals could be added to reflect palliative/hospice care provision. For example:
  - Patients and care partners will use strategies to facilitate the patient's ability to communicate care preferences or concerns and to maintain a social connection for end-of-life care.
  - Patient and care partners will demonstrate eating, drinking, or swallowing strategies that support patient comfort and preference associated with end-of-life care plans.

Table 2–4. Writing Palliative Care Speech-Language Pathology Goals

This table provides a template for creating participation-based palliative care speech-language pathology goals. It is provided as a model for goal creation; additional types of outcomes and purposes can also be addressed through development of authentic treatment goals set with the patient and their caregivers.

Domain	Targeted Outcome of SLP Intervention	Palliative Care Purpose
Communication and cognition	Patient will . . .	
	Use augmentative communication strategies	. . . to facilitate social/emotional connection with family
	Communicate using visual aids	. . . to communicate needs and preferences for end-of-life care
	Increase use of vocal/articulatory strategies	. . . to communicate status for symptom management
		. . . to express spiritual or emotional concerns
		. . . to engage in chosen activities or end-of-life goals
	Care partners will . . .	
	Use conversation partner strategies	. . . to include the patient in decision making for care
	Use voice amplifier during care conversations	. . . to maintain patient's awareness of goals of care OR to maintain social/ emotional connection
	Obtain and use alerting device	. . . to enable patient to alert care provider for immediate care needs
	Use augmentative communication aids	. . . to enable patient to participate in spiritual/emotional support
Eating, drinking, and swallowing	Patient will . . .	
	Use augmentative communication strategies	. . . to select preferred foods for pleasure eating
	Communicate using visual aids	. . . to improve patient understanding of options for nutrition, hydration, or medication intake
	Utilize [specific dysphagia] strategies	. . . to facilitate ease of eating and drinking for comfort at meals
	Care partners will . . .	
	Use augmentative communication strategies	. . . to support positive mealtime interactions with patient
	Utilize strategies	. . . to provide optimal oral care

THE ROLE OF SPIRITUALITY IN END-OF-LIFE CARE

Most deaths in the United States occur in institutions (e.g., hospitals and nursing homes), and among people who die in health care settings, more than one-third report insufficient emotional support (Teno et al., 2004). Emotional support may come from several sources, including social workers, psychologists, nurses, physicians, or spiritual care staff or volunteers. Spiritual care is integral to palliative care for many patients and families. Studies show that the inclusion of spiritual care is associated with a higher quality of life for patients as they near the EoL (Koper et al., 2019; Soroka et al., 2019). In the context of palliative care, spiritual care services offer broad support as patients and families grapple with acceptance of their circumstances; seek support for reconciliation with family, friends, or personal relationships to faith; explore existential issues, including finding meaning in life and death; and discuss EoL wishes and/or after-death planning including funeral arrangements (Balboni et al., 2010; El Nawawi et al., 2012; Koper et al., 2019). In the United States, spiritual care is typically provided by staff, volunteer pastors, chaplains, or spiritual care coordinators. Although hospice and palliative care services consider spiritual care providers as core health care team members, spiritual needs may be unmet or delayed for patients because of institutional or personal barriers.

Patients who practice a nonmainstream religion may not have access to hospital-based staff who can offer spiritual care that aligns with their faith and beliefs. Similarly, patients who hold spiritual beliefs but do not practice a particular religion may not promptly be referred for spiritual care services. Even when spiritual care is offered, patients do not always welcome spiritual support and may refuse such services for various reasons (Soroka et al., 2019). For example, patients or their families may reject spiritual care due to differences within the family about religious or spiritual practices. Such discordance can limit access to support for the patient, the family, or both.

Role of the SLP in Spiritual Care

Physicians and other health care providers have often been explicitly taught to avoid discussion of religion in clinical contexts. As a result, clinicians may need instruction about responding appropriately to a patient's spiritual needs (Collier et al., 2021). SLP training is no exception (Kirsh et al., 2001).

Very few studies have directly addressed the role of the SLP in spiritual care. However, many authors have explored the role of spiritual care under broader areas such as client-centered care (Mathisen et al., 2015; Spillers, 2010), EoL care (Chahda et al., 2017; Groher & Groger, 2012; Rivers et al., 2009), and cultural and linguistic diversity (Cheng, 2009; Ezrati-Vinacour & Weinstein, 2011). Mathisen and Threats (2018) suggest several reasons SLPs should include spiritual care in their practice, including the role of religion or spiritual care in patient-centered practice and data that demonstrate improved outcomes, including quality of life and patient awareness of their clinical status. SLPs may be asked to support communication or eating, drinking, and swallowing for patient access to spiritual care.

Religion and spirituality often play a prominent role in EoL care, thus SLPs must be prepared to understand and support this need. When appropriate, spiritual assessment should be included within clinical practice, and all interventions for communication, cognition, and swallowing should account for individual patients' spiritual beliefs.

Suggestions for SLPs to Include Spiritual Care in Their Practice

- Be sensitive to and aware of the importance of spiritual care for patients and their families.

- Build awareness of evidence that religious and spiritual beliefs impact the patient experience and contribute to clinical decision making.

- Include religious or spirituality screening in intake assessments.

- Learn how to refer patients for spiritual support (see also Chapter 4 and Table 4–3).

- Ensure communication support for those near the EoL includes emotional well-being, religion, and spirituality when desired.

- Ensure that feeding and dysphagia support for those near the EoL accounts for spiritual beliefs and needs around food and drink.

- Ensure that any decisional aids used or recommended account for religious and spiritual beliefs.

OVERCOMING BARRIERS TO SPEECH-LANGUAGE PATHOLOGY INVOLVEMENT IN END-OF-LIFE CARE

Western cultures frequently avoid the topic of death and dying (Gawande, 2014; Mannix, 2018; Pascoe et al., 2018; Puri, 2019; Rivers et al., 2009; Roe & Leslie, 2010; Stead & McDonnell, 2015). Sociocultural discomfort with death and dying extends to Western medicine and clinical training programs across professions (Gawande, 2014; Mannix, 2018). It is atypical for graduate programs in speech-language pathology to include instruction about the role of the SLP in the care of patients who are dying and how the focus of care differs from typical (re)habilitative approaches that are the centerpiece of SLP training (Stead et al., 2023). The absence of explicit training for new SLPs creates a lack of clarity about the role of the SLP in EoL care and is a barrier to optimizing care for patients with life-limiting conditions. Most often SLPs learn and work within a model of habilitation or rehabilitation with a focus on maximizing functional skills. Exposure to the ways in which SLPs can support patients when function is expected to decline fosters SLPs' understanding of their role with this population. On reflection, it is not difficult to see why ensuring access to communication and supporting eating, drinking, and swallowing are essential aspects of patients' care and contributes to their sense of control and well-being.

Systems and Institutional Barriers to Speech-Language Services

Systems structures in hospice and palliative medicine typically consult SLPs as an adjunct service rather than the SLP being genuinely integrated as a care team member (Misra et al., 2018; Roe & Leslie, 2010; Wallace, 2013). SLPs are consulted on an as-needed basis, and this referral model relies on the knowledge and insight of an individual nurse, social worker, physician, or another member of the palliative care team to identify when a patient could benefit from speech-language services. When these referrals occur, dysphagia is the most likely focus (Hawksley et al., 2017).

Physicians, nurses, social workers, other team members, and families often lack awareness about the direct and indirect services SLPs can provide (Wallace, 2013). As a result, it is not uncommon for SLPs to encounter professionals who believe that individuals nearing the EoL cannot benefit from rehabilitative services. This perception occasionally emerges for patients with a do not resuscitate (DNR) order within rehabilitation settings.

Overcoming Institutional Barriers to Speech-Language Pathology Services at the End of Life

SLPs can contribute to institutional and systems change in several ways. A powerful tool is direct contact with core hospice and palliative care team members to identify interest in offering support to them and their patients. These teams can benefit from information about how to make a referral for speech-language pathology services that will ensure their patients are connected with an SLP who is prepared to support the particular needs of patients with life-limiting conditions.

Institutional change can happen in many ways. Although each clinician's context differs, a core set of driving questions can begin a pathway to change: (a) If there were no obstacles or barriers, what is the best EoL care we could offer here? (b) What changes would improve

---

Answer the Following Questions to Begin Creating Institutional Change

- Who are the key people involved?
  - Who are your allies?
  - How can you build on strengths and relationships?
- How can you obtain buy-in?
  - What are the goals of the key people involved?
  - What value can you add to help meet those goals?
- How can you contribute to change?
  - What do you need to *know* to institute these changes?
  - What knowledge or skills do you need to develop?
  - What do you need to *do* to institute these changes?
  - What are the barriers?
- How will you know the goals have been accomplished?
  - What data should you or your employer gather? (e.g., baseline rates of referral, diagnostic groups served, clinical outcomes, or quality improvement metrics such as patient/family satisfaction data)

- How can you sustain change?
  - Build institutional awareness. For example, offer to give a grand rounds talk or in-service training for the palliative or hospice team and/or develop an institutional newsletter or web-based article.
  - Encourage institutional recognition of quality EoL care through clinical service awards or spotlight clinical excellence.
  - Disseminate programmatic changes within the profession of speech-language pathology through institutional discussions at the department level.
  - Identify colleagues at other institutions to serve as mutual resources and support.
  - Start a regional interest group or journal club.
  - Report research through presentations, special interest groups, and/or professional journal articles.

EoL care here? and (c) What are the barriers to initiating these changes? Once these foundational questions are addressed, clinicians and institutions can address barriers to effective service. The Institutional Change Box provides example questions to help clinicians initiate the process of change within a setting.

As the SLP works to build professional relationships, it is often valuable to request to join a team meeting to follow up on a given referral or to observe. Through participation, the SLP will likely identify other patients and families who could benefit from assessment and/or intervention. If the team is open to an offer of a brief in-service presentation or workshop, the SLP can build the knowledge and skills of core team members (Pollens, 2012). Some of these constructs can seem almost self-evident to SLPs, but it is expected that patients, families, and other health professionals use terms such as "speech" and "language" interchangeably. If the core team members

who conduct patient intake and ongoing assessment build their knowledge of communication, cognition, and swallowing and understand how an SLP can assist them in the care of their patients, they are more likely to develop a pattern of appropriate referrals for speech-language pathology services and support.

When referrals arise, the SLP should ensure excellent communication of recommendations and outcomes to the care team. If the referral is limited to one domain of concern, the SLP should note any other areas of function that could contribute to the patient's well-being. For example, if the patient is referred for swallowing and the SLP notes the patient would benefit from voice amplification, the SLP should include that recommendation. As the value of speech-language pathology services for patients who are nearing the EoL is demonstrated, the SLP is likely to become a more integral part of the care team with earlier identification of those patients who experience barriers to communication and/or eating, drinking, and swallowing (Pollens, 2012).

Sample Constructs of Communication, Cognition, and Swallowing to Enhance the Knowledge and Skills of Other Health Professionals

- the distinction between language comprehension and language expression
- speech production and intelligibility
- descriptors of voice quality
- hearing and its role in speech and language
- cognitive constructs
- eating, drinking, and swallowing best practices
- sample intervention strategies such as low-technology alternative communication boards

---

SELF-CARE FOR THE CLINICIAN IN EOL CARE

Clinicians who serve patients and families during the process of dying report joy and satisfaction associated with this work (Kirkland, 2017; Mannix, 2018; Twycross, 1997); nevertheless, the experience of suffering and death and ongoing experiences of loss pose risks for negative impacts of chronic stress on all clinical professionals.

Regardless of the setting, clinicians benefit from the knowledge of what burnout is, the contributors to burnout, and the steps to avoid burnout. Although the term "burnout" is often used casually, there is a specific definition that cuts across three dimensions: (a) exhaustion (physical and/or emotional), (b) low sense of efficacy, and (c) cynicism (Maslach et al., 2001). Risk factors for true burnout include perfectionism, difficulty setting clear boundaries, a high need for recognition and/or pleasing people, and feeling irreplaceable. Symptoms of burnout are both physical and behavioral. Physical symptoms include chronic headaches, gastrointestinal symptoms, personal neglect, and/or physical exhaustion, while behavioral symptoms may include sleep disturbance, depression, substance abuse, and/or anxiety (De Hert, 2020).

Clinicians are often advised to engage in self-care, which is overly simplified to such things as taking a warm bath or a walk. In reality, self-care requires ongoing thoughtful prevention and self-awareness strategies that occur alongside a shared responsibility of the employer. Employers are responsible for engaging in meaningful support systems for employees, including stress management, paid days off, and flexibility to take time in the immediate aftermath of challenging clinical situations. Ideally, employee wellness programs and/or health coverage will include mental health and counseling services.

Clinical employees should have the opportunity to engage in meaningful discussions of their work with colleagues, support for continuing education, and recognition of their work and service. Employers that engage in transparent communication offer positive feedback and explicitly support well-functioning teams that contribute to longevity and employee well-being (De Hert, 2020). High-functioning teams provide collective support through shared understanding (Kirkland, 2017; Sharp, 1995).

SLPs who work on contract or as consultants to teams should be aware of the increased risk of stress or burnout due to isolation. SLPs who work in relative isolation as a contract service provider or private practice hold additional responsibilities for self-monitoring and self-care. SLPs at elevated risk can implement proactive strategies such as consistent engagement with other care team members. For example, a hospice team may not require the SLP to attend team meetings as a noncore team member. However, elective participation can contribute to collaboration and shared understanding across team members who serve as a source of support. Increased visibility of the SLP in the team context will likely contribute to increased utilization of speech-language services as team members learn more about the value of communication and SLP support for patients, families, and members of the professional team.

SLPs who work in end-of-life care can and should identify others in their community, region, country, or internationally who also work in this area. Such professional collaboration enhances the knowledge and skills of all professionals, becomes a source of professional support, and ultimately improves services and the quality of clinical care.

CONCLUSIONS

Hospice and palliative care focus on symptom management and patient-centered goals of care that best support the patient's quality of life goals. Nearly all patients experience communication, cognitive, and/or eating, drinking, or swallowing problems as they near the EoL. Communication is essential for patients to convey symptoms and the effectiveness of symptom management strategies, to set goals of care, and to engage in social/emotional and spiritual conversations with family, members of the care team, and others. Changes in eating, drinking, and swallowing can be scary to patients who experience weight loss, gastrointestinal distress, coughing, and other symptoms. Caregivers also observe these changes in food and fluid intake and may feel responsible for what they perceive as inadequate care. The SLP can provide valuable strategies, tools, and counseling to optimize patient care and to lessen caregiver distress while the patient is dying and after the patient's death.

The SLP is well prepared to provide comprehensive information to patients, families, and health care professionals about communication, cognition, and swallowing function based on a careful clinical assessment informed by patient preference. SLPs may develop specific, direct or indirect intervention plans to support communication function, train communication partners, or consult with members of the professional team to keep patients' communication, eating, and cognitive needs at the forefront.

REFERENCES

Accreditation Council for Graduate Medical Education. (n.d.). https://www.acgme.org/

American Academy of Hospice and Palliative Medicine. (n.d.). https://aahpm.org/

American Speech-Language-Hearing Association. (n.d.). *End of life issues in speech-language pathology.* https://www.asha.org/slp/clinical/endoflife/

Balboni, T. A., Paulk, M. E., Balboni, M. J., Phelps, A. C., Loggers, E. T., Wright, A. A., . . . Prigerson, H. G. (2010). Provision of spiritual care to patients with advanced cancer: Associations with medical care and quality of life near death. *Journal of Clinical Oncology, 28*(3), 445.

Balboni, T. A., Vanderwerker, L. C., Block, S. D., Paulk, M. E., Lathan, C. S., Peteet, J. R., & Prigerson, H. G. (2007). Religiousness and spiritual support among advanced cancer patients and associations with end-of-life treatment preferences and quality of life. *Journal of Clinical Oncology, 25*(5), 555.

Bogaardt, H., Veerbeek, L., Kelly, K., van der Heide, A., van Zuylen, L., & Speyer, R. (2015). Swallowing problems at the end of the palliative phase: Incidence and severity in 164 unsedated patients. *Dysphagia, 30,* 144–151.

Brownlee, A., & Bruening, L. M. (2012). Methods of communication at end of life for the person with amyotrophic lateral sclerosis. *Topics in Language Disorders, 32,* 168–185. http://doi.org/10.1097/TLD.0b013e31825616ef

Castro, C. M., Wilson, C., Wang, F., & Schillinger, D. (2007). Babel babble: Physicians' use of unclarified medical jargon with patients. *American Journal of Health Behavior, 31*(1), S85–S95.

Center for Medicare Services. (2021). *Medicare benefit policy manual. Chapter 9—Coverage of hospice services under hospital insurance.* https://www.cms.gov/Regulations-and-Guidance/Guidance/Manuals/Downloads/bp102c09.pdf

Chahda, L., Mathisen, B. A., & Carey, L. B. (2017). The role of speech-language pathologists in adult palliative care. *International Journal of Speech-Language Pathology, 19*(1), 58–68.

Chandregowda, A., Stierwalt, J. A., & Clark, H. M. (2021). Facilitating end-of-life interaction between patients with severe communication impairment and their families. *Perspectives of the ASHA Special Interest Groups, 6*(3), 649–653. https://doi.org/10.1044/2021_PERSP-20-00282

Cheng, L. R. L. (2009). Creating an optimal language learning environment: A focus on family and culture. *Communication Disorders Quarterly, 30*(2), 69–76.

Childers, J. W., Back, A. L., Tulsky, J. A., & Arnold, R. M. (2017). REMAP: A framework for goals of care conversations. *Journal of Oncology Practice, 13*(10), e844–e850.

Collier, K. M., James, C. A., Saint, S., & Howell, J. (2021). The role of spirituality and religion in physician and trainee wellness. *Journal of General Internal Medicine, 36*(10), 3199–3201.

Collins, C. A. (2022). "There's this big fear around palliative care because it's connected to death and dying": A qualitative exploration of the perspectives of undergraduate students on the role of the speech and language therapist in palliative care. *Palliative Medicine, 36*(1), 171–180.

Connolly, T., Coats, H., DeSanto, K., & Jones, J. (2021). The experience of uncertainty for patients, families and healthcare providers in post-stroke palliative and end-of-life care: A qualitative meta-synthesis. *Age and Ageing*, *50*(2), 534–545.

De Hert, S. (2020). Burnout in healthcare workers: Prevalence, impact, and preventive strategies. *Local and Regional Anesthesia*, *13*, 171–183. http://doi.org/10.2147/LRA.S240564

Detering, K. M., Hancock, A. D., Reade, M. C., & Silvester, W. (2010). The impact of advance care planning on end of life care in elderly patients: Randomized controlled trial. *The British Medical Journal*, *340*, C1345. http://doi.org/10.1136/bmj.c1345

Dunne, K. (2005). Effective communication in palliative care. *Nursing Standard (through 2013)*, *20*(13), 57.

Egan, K. (2017). *On living*. Riverhead Books.

El Nawawi, N. M., Balboni, M. J., & Balboni, T. A. (2012). Palliative care and spiritual care: The crucial role of spiritual care in the care of patients with advanced illness. *Current Opinion in Supportive and Palliative Care*, *6*(2), 269–274.

Eubanks, C. F., Burckell, L. A., & Goldfried, M. R. (2018). Clinical consensus strategies to repair ruptures in the therapeutic alliance. *Journal of Psychotherapy Integration*, *28*(1), 60.

Ezrati-Vinacour, R., & Weinstein, N. (2011). A dialogue among various cultures and its manifestation in stuttering therapy. *Journal of Fluency Disorders*, *36*(3), 174–185.

Fallowfield, L., & Jenkins, V. (2004). Communicating sad, bad, and difficult news in medicine. *The Lancet*, *363*(9405), 312–319.

Garrett, K., Happ, M., Costello, J., & Fried-Oken, M. (2007). AAC in the intensive care unit. In D. Beukelman, K. Garrett, & K. Yorkston (Eds.), *Augmentative communication strategies for adults with acute or chronic medical conditions* (pp. 17–59). Brookes.

Gawande, A. (2014). *Being mortal: Medicine and what matters in the end*. Picador.

Girgis, A., & Sanson-Fisher, R. W. (1998). Breaking bad news. 1: Current best advice for clinicians. *Behavioral Medicine*, *24*(2), 53–59.

Glare, P., Walsh, D., & Sheehan, D. (2016). The adverse effects of morphine: A prospective survey of common symptoms during repeated dosing for chronic cancer pain. *American Journal of Hospice and Palliative Medicine*, *23*(3), 229–235.

Gold, R., & Gold, A. (2018). Delivering bad news: Attitudes, feelings, and practice characteristics among speech-language pathologists. *American Journal of Speech-Language Pathology*, *27*(1), 108–122. https://doi.org/10.1044/2017_AJSLP-17-0045

Gonella, S., Campagna, S., Basso, I., Grazia De Marinis, M., & Di Giulio, P. (2019). Mechanisms by which end-of-life communication influences palliative-oriented care in nursing homes: A scoping review. *Patient Education and Counseling*, *102*(12), 2134–2144.

Graham, S., & Brookey, J. (2008). Do patients understand? *The Permanente Journal*, *12*(3), 67–69. https://doi.org/10.7812/tpp/07-144

Groher, M. E., & Groher, T. P. (2012). When safe oral feeding is threatened: End-of-life options and decisions. *Topics in Language Disorders*, *32*(2), 149–167.

Gustafsson, A., Skogsberg, J., & Rejnö, Å. (2021). Oral health plays second fiddle in palliative care: An interview study with registered nurses in home healthcare. *BMC Palliative Care*, *20*(1), 1–11.

Hawksley, R., Ludlow, F., Buttimer, H., & Bloch, S. (2017). Communication disorders in palliative care: Investigating the views, attitudes, and beliefs of speech and language therapists. *International Journal of Palliative Nursing*, *23*(11), 543–551.

Health Canada. (2018). *Framework on palliative care in Canada*. https://www.canada.ca/content/dam/hc-sc/documents/services/health-care-system/reports-publications/palliative-care/framework-palliative-care-canada/framework-palliative-care-canada.pdf

Holland, A. L., & Nelson, R. L. (2018). *Counseling in communication disorders: A wellness perspective* (3rd ed.). Plural.

Hong Kong Institute of Speech Therapists. (2021). *Guideline for speech therapy service in residential care homes for the elderly*. https://hkist.org.hk/wp-content/uploads/2022/09/Doc.-No.-26-HKIST-Guideline-for-ST-service-in-RCHEs-v1.pdf

Javier, N. S., & Montagnini, M. L. (2011). Rehabilitation of the hospice and palliative care patient. *Journal of Palliative Medicine, 14*(5), 638–648.

Kagan, A. (1998). Supported conversation for adults with aphasia: Methods and resources for training conversation partners. *Aphasiology, 12*(9), 816–830.

Kessels, R. P. (2003). Patients' memory for medical information. *Journal of the Royal Society of Medicine, 96*(5), 219–222. https://www.ncbi.nlm.nih.gov/pmc/articles/PMC539473/

Kirkland, K. B. (2017). Finding joy in practice: Cocreation in palliative care. *Journal of the American Medical Association, 317*(20), 2065–2066. http://doi.org/10.1001/jama.2017.1109

Kirsh, B., Dawson, D., Antolikova, S., & Reynolds, L. (2001). Developing awareness of spirituality in occupational therapy students: Are our curricula up to the task? *Occupational Therapy International, 8*(2), 119–125.

Koper, I., Pasman, H. R. W., Schweitzer, B. P., Kuin, A., & Onwuteaka-Philipsen, B. D. (2019). Spiritual care at the end of life in the primary care setting: Experiences from spiritual caregivers—A mixed methods study. *BMC Palliative Care, 18*(1), 1–10.

Krikheli, L., Mathisen, B. A., & Carey, L. B. (2018). Speech–language pathology in paediatric palliative care: A scoping review of role and practice. *International Journal of Speech-Language Pathology, 20*(5), 541–553.

Levin, T. T., Moreno, B., Silvester, W., & Kissane, D. W. (2010). End-of-life communication in the intensive care unit. *General Hospital Psychiatry, 32*(4), 433–442.

Luterman, D. M. (2016). *Counseling persons with communication disorders and their families* (6th ed.). Pro-Ed.

Maeda, K., & Akagi, J. (2014). Oral care may reduce pneumonia in the tube-fed elderly: A preliminary study. *Dysphagia, 29*(5), 616–621.

Magnani, C., Mastroianni, C., Giannarelli, D., Stefanelli, M. C., Di Cienzo, V., Valerioti, T., & Casale, G. (2019). Oral hygiene care in patients with advanced disease: An essential measure to improve oral cavity conditions and symptom management. *American Journal of Hospice and Palliative Medicine*, *36*(9), 815–819.

Manderson, L., & Warren, N. (2010). The art of (re)learning to walk: Trust on the rehabilitation ward. *Qualitative Health Research, 20*(10), 1418–1432.

Mannix, K. (2018). *With the end in mind: Dying, death, and wisdom in an age of denial.* Little, Brown, Spark.

Maslach, C., Schaufeli, W. B., & Leiter, M. P. (2001). Job burnout. *Annual Review of Psychology, 52*, 97–422. http://doi.org/10.1146/annurev.psych.52.1.397

Mathisen, B., Carey, L. B., Carey-Sargeant, C. L., Webb, G., Millar, C., & Krikheli, L. (2015). Religion, spirituality and speech-language pathology: A viewpoint for ensuring patient-centered holistic care. *Journal of Religion and Health, 54*(6), 2309–2323.

Mathisen, B., & Threats, T. (2018). Speech-language pathology and spiritual care. In L. Carey & B. Mathisen (Eds.), *Spiritual care for allied health practice* (pp. 22–54). Jessica Kingsley Publishers.

McCann, R. M., Hall, W. J., & Groth-Junker, A. (1994). Comfort care for terminally ill patients: The appropriate use of nutrition and hydration. *Journal of the American Medical Association, 272*(16), 1263–1266.

Minton, M. E., Isaacson, M. J., Varilek, B. M., Stadick, J. L., & O'Connell-Persaud, S. (2018). A willingness to go there: Nurses and spiritual care. *Journal of Clinical Nursing, 27*(1–2), 173–181.

Misra, S., Ashford, M., & Leyhew, B. (2018). "Is NPO the only option?" An innovative research-based framework for oral intake recommendations in the seriously ill. The Annual Assembly of the American Academy of Hospice and Palliative Medicine and the Hospice and Palliative Nurses Association Education Schedule with Abstracts. *Journal of Pain and Symptom Management, 55*(2), 548–653.

Morrison, R. S., Meier, D. E., & Arnold, R. M. (2021). What's wrong with advance care planning? *Journal of the American Medical Association, 326*(16), 1575–1576. http://doi.org/10.1001/jama.2021.16430

National Consensus Project for Quality Palliative Care. (2018). *Clinical guidelines for quality palliative care* (4th ed). National Coalition for Hospice and Palliative Care.

Ngo-Metzger, Q., August, K. J., Srinivasan, M., Liao, S., & Meyskens, F. L., Jr. (2008). End-of-life care: Guidelines for patient-centered communication. *American Family Physician, 77*(2), 167–174.

O'Reilly, A. C., & Walshe, M. (2015). Perspectives on the role of the speech and language therapist in palliative care: An international survey. *Palliative Medicine, 29*(8), 756–761.

Pitt, M. B., & Hendrickson, M. A. (2020). Eradicating jargon-oblivion—A proposed classification system of medical jargon. *Journal of General Internal Medicine, 35*(6), 1861–1864.

Pascoe, A., Breen, L. J., & Cocks, N. (2018). What is needed to prepare speech pathologists to work in adult palliative care? *International Journal of Language & Communication Disorders, 53*(3), 542–549. https://doi.org/10.1111/1460-6984.12367

Pollens, R. (2004). Role of the speech-language pathologist in palliative hospice care. *Journal of Palliative Medicine, 7*, 694–702. http://doi.org/10.1089/jpm.2004.7.694

Pollens, R. (2012). Integrating speech-language pathology services in palliative end-of-life care. *Topics in Language Disorders, 32*, 137–148. http://doi.org/10.1097/TLD.0b013e3182543533

Pollens, R. (2020). Facilitating client ability to communicate in palliative end-of-life care: Impact of speech-language pathologists. *Topics in Language Disorders, 40*(3), 264–277.

Pollens, R., Chahda, L., Freeman-Sanderson, A., Lalonde Myers, E., & Mathison, B. (2021). Supporting crucial conversations: Speech-language pathology intervention in palliative end-of-life care. *Journal of Palliative Medicine, 24*(7), 969–970.

Pollens, R., & Lynn, M. (2011). Social work and speech pathology: Supporting communication in palliative care. *Oxford textbook of palliative social work* (pp. 483–487). Oxford University Press.

Pound, L. (1936). American euphemisms for dying, death, and burial: An anthology. *American Speech, 11*(3), 195–202.

Puri, S. (2019). *That good night: Life and medicine in the eleventh hour*. Constable.

Rimmer, A. (2014). Doctors must avoid jargon when talking to patients, Royal College says. *British Medical Journal, 348*, g4131. https://www.doi.org/10.1136/bmj.g4131

Rivers, K. O., Perkins, R. A., & Carson, C. P. (2009). Perceptions of speech-pathology and audiology students concerning death and dying: A preliminary study. *International Journal of Language & Communication Disorders, 44*(1), 98–111.

Roe, J. W., & Leslie, P. (2010). Beginning of the end? Ending the therapeutic relationship in palliative care. *International Journal of Speech-Language Pathology, 12*(4), 304–308.

Royal College of Speech and Language Therapists. (2023, January 20). *End of life care overview.* https://www.rcslt.org/speech-and-language-therapy/clinical-information/end-of-life-care-overview/

Santiago-Palma, J., & Payne, R. (2001). Palliative care and rehabilitation. *Cancer, 92*, 1049–1052.

Saunders, C. M., & Clark, D. (2006). *Cicely Saunders: Selected writings 1958–2004*. Oxford University Press.

Schleinich, M., Warren, S., Nekolaichuk, C., Kaasa, R., & Watanabe, S. (2008). Palliative care rehabilitation survey: A pilot study of patients' priorities for rehabilitation goals. *Palliative Medicine, 22*, 822–830. http://doi.org/10.1177/0269216308096526

Schofield, C., Bennett, R., Orloff, C., & Devalia, U. (2022). Children's hospices: An opportunity to put the mouth back in the body. *British Dental Journal, 22*, 1–6. http://doi.org/10.1038/s41415-022-4926-y

Sharp, H. M. (1995). Ethical decision-making in interdisciplinary team care. *The Cleft Palate-Craniofacial Journal, 32*(6), 495–499.

Sharp, H. M., & Payne, S. K. (1999). Caring for patients at the end of life. In P. A. Sullivan & A. M. Guilford (Eds.), *Swallowing intervention in oncology*. (pp. 329–342), Singular Publishing.

Soileau, K., & Elster, N. (2018). The hospice patient's right to oral care: Making time for the mouth. *Journal of Palliative Care, 33*(2), 65–69. http://doi.org/10.1177/0825859718763283

Soroka, J. T., Collins, L. A., Creech, G., Kutcher, G. R., Menne, K. R., & Petzel, B. L. (2019). Spiritual care at the end of life: Does educational intervention focused on a broad definition of spirituality increase utilization of chaplain spiritual support in hospice?. *Journal of Palliative Medicine, 22*(8), 939–944.

Spillers, C. S. (2010). Spiritual dimensions of the clinical relationship. In R. J. Fourie (Ed.), *Therapeutic processes for communication disorders* (pp. 245–260). Psychology Press.

Stead, A., Dirks, K., Fryer, M., & Wong, S. (2020). Training future clinicians for work in palliative care. *Topics in Language Disorders, 20*(3), 233–247. https://doi.org/10.1097/TLD.00000000 00000219

Stead, A., Haynie, S., & Vinson, M. (2023). Teaching end-of-life care in speech-pathology graduate programs: A tutorial. *Teaching and Learning in Communication Sciences and Disorders, 7*(1). https://doi.org/10.30707/TLCSD7 .1.1675490380.883534

Stead, A., & McDonnell, C. (2015). End of life care: An opportunity. *Perspectives in Gerontology, 20*(1), 12–15. https://doi.org/10.1044/ gero20.1.12

Sterling, L., Axline, R., & Ragland, P. (2013). Food for thought. *Perspectives of the ASHA Special Interest Groups, 22*(1), 32–37. https://doi .org/10.1044/sasd22.1.32

Teno, J. M., Clarridge, B. R., Casey, V., Welch, L. C., Wetle, T., Shield, R., & Mor, V. (2004). Family perspectives on end-of-life care at the last place of care. *JAMA, 291*(1), 88–93.

Toner, M. A., & Shadden, B. B. (2012). End of life: An overview. *Topics in Language Disorders, 32*(2), 111–118.

Twycross, R. G. (1981). Rehabilitation in terminal cancer patients. *International Rehabilitation Medicine, 3*, 135–144.

Twycross, R. (1997). The joy of death. *The Lancet, 350*(9094), S11120.

Venkatasalu, M. R., Murang, Z. R., Ramasamy, D. T. R., & Dhaliwal, J. S. (2020). Oral health problems among palliative and terminally ill patients: An integrated systematic review. *BMC Oral Health, 20*, 79. http://doi.org/10.1186/ s12903-020-01075-w

Wallace, G. (2013). Speech-language pathology: Enhancing quality of life for individuals approaching death. *Perspectives on Gerontology, 18*(3), 112–120.

Williams, A. M. (2018). Education, training, and mentorship of caregivers of Canadians experiencing a life-limiting illness. *Journal of Palliative Medicine, 21*(Suppl. 1), S45–S49. https://doi .org/10.1089/jpm.2017.0393

World Health Organization. (2016). *Planning and implementing palliative care services: A guide for programme managers.* WHO Press.

World Health Organization. (2022). *Palliative care.* https://www.who.int/news-room/fact-sheets/ detail/palliative-care

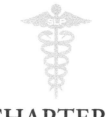

CHAPTER 3

The Role of Patient Preferences in End-of-Life Care

Helen Sharp

> *"To know the patient that has the disease is more important than to know the disease that the patient has."*—Sir William Osler

INTRODUCTION

Patients at every age and stage of life have a fundamental need and right to understand their health status and to communicate their basic physiologic needs. As patients near the end of life (EoL), it is vital to convey basic care needs and preferences for care and to communicate with their health care providers, community of spiritual advisors, friends, and loved ones. When there are barriers to communication, speech-language pathologists (SLPs) can assess and intervene to support communication (see Chapter 4).

Ongoing attention to communication is essential because the trajectory toward EoL nearly always involves decisions for patients and their caregivers (Anderson et al., 2019). Each patient's situation differs medically, socially, psychologically, and spiritually. Individuals' decisions are strongly influenced by

their lived experience, religious or spiritual beliefs, values, culture, individual goals and preferences, and the preferences of family and friends who form the individual's community. In the context of this variability, the role of every clinician is to set aside assumptions, listen deeply, and recognize the patient's individual needs and those of their loved ones (Sprik & Gentile, 2020). SLPs are particularly well equipped to advocate for patients to ensure communication with medical providers, family members, friends, and others is optimized.

In this chapter, we will explore why it is essential for each member of the health care team to partner with patients and families through a process of shared decision making. Shared decision making and strong clinician–patient relationships create trust and allow for meaningful, informed decision making that upholds the patient's values and preferences. In the context of interprofessional team care, SLPs have the knowledge and skills to support ongoing participation in decision making for as long as possible. To do so, SLPs must be familiar with the construct of informed consent and be able to identify the cognitive and communication skills required for patients to demonstrate they have the capacity to make informed decisions. SLPs should also be familiar with how to approach decision making when adults can no longer make decisions for themselves. We will also examine the role of children and adolescents in decision making about their care.

THE ROLE OF SHARED DECISION MAKING IN CLINICAL CARE

Respect for an individual's decisions to accept or refuse health care or to participate in research is a core principle of bioethics referred to as respect for autonomy (Beauchamp & Childress, 2019). Respect for autonomy (self-determination) is a cornerstone of contemporary Western health care and is well codified in U.S. law (Cruzan v. Director, Missouri Department of Health, 1990; Schloendorff v. Society of New York Hospital, 1914) and the literature in bioethics (e.g., Beauchamp & Childress, 2019; Jonsen et al., 2022; Lo, 2019; Macauley, 2018). When a health professional seeks a patient's consent to conduct an assessment, initiate treatment, or engage in research, the assumption that a patient has a right to agree or refuse is grounded in the principle of respect for autonomy.

To act autonomously and make informed decisions, patients rely on health professionals' honesty and ability to convey understandable and accurate information. Therefore, the principle of respect for autonomy overlaps with truth telling, another core principle of bioethics (principle of veracity) (Back et al., 2009; Beauchamp & Childress, 2019).

> **The Four Principles of Bioethics**
> (Beauchamp & Childress, 2019)
>
> - Respect for autonomy: the clinician's duty to respect the patient's right to self-determination
> - Beneficence: the clinician's duty to act in the interest of the patient and maximize the patient's welfare
> - Nonmaleficence: the clinician's duty to do no harm
> - Justice: the clinician's duty to provide fair and equitable care

Shared Decision Making in Clinical Care

Shared decision making in clinical care balances respect for the patient's preference with the reasonable options available to the health care professional or health care team. Shared decision making is achieved through an ongoing commitment to partnership between clinician and patient that is reflected through listening to the patient's goals, values, and preferences that embed the patient's cultural, religious, spiritual, and community perspectives and allow for meaningful, individualized patient education and discussion (Anderson et al., 2019; Janssen & MacLeod, 2010; Jonsen et al., 2022; Linebarger et al., 2022). Shared decision making honors a patient's right to self-determination through the process of informed consent or its equal counterpart, informed refusal.

Although shared decision making is the ideal, in practice, patients often experience parentalism in their care (Macauley, 2018). Parentalism (also called paternalism) aligns with the "doctor knows best" approach to decision making that places the health professional in a dominant role and the patient as subordinate. For example, when a lump or lesion is identified, the patient hears "We *need* to get a CT scan or MRI," "We *need* to take a biopsy," or "We *need* to take a blood draw to assess your lab values." This clinician-dominated approach often reflects a well-intentioned desire to act in the patient's best interest (principle of beneficence) (Beauchamp & Childress, 2019). However, ultimately a clinician's unilateral decision on behalf of a patient is inherently prone to error and contributes to the power imbalance between clinicians and patients.

A potential danger of a parentalistic approach is the appearance that a patient has acted autonomously and given consent, simply because the patient did not question or refuse at any step (Macauley, 2018). However, the requirements of informed consent have not been met if the patient does not know or understand the broader purpose of the proposed medical interventions. If the patient is given "We *need* . . . " statements without alternatives or adequate information about the purpose, risks, and benefits to these recommendations, then they have not given informed consent.

In a paternalistic model of care, the patient or their family caregivers may be invited to discuss their preferences, state their goals of care, or make choices only when decisions become complex or uncertain. From the patient/family perspective, this shift can be abrupt and is likely to be perceived as abandonment or an abdication of the clinician's responsibilities. Surviving family members identify such shifts in responsibility as a source of stress and guilt long after the patient's death (Wendler & Rid, 2011). Shared decision making should not be introduced when a patient experiences a health crisis or when decision making becomes complicated. Rather, the practice of shared decision making through-

out the trajectory of care strengthens clinician–patient relationships, prepares patients and families to manage complex decisions, improves outcomes, reduces inequities, and reduces stress for surrogate decision makers (National Health Service (NHS), 2019; Sahgal et al., 2021). Ideally, clinicians should engage patients in shared decision making across every clinical encounter.

Shared decision making relies on clinician expertise and guidance, truth telling, clear communication, and respect for the individual patient's preferences and values (Back et al., 2009; Mannix, 2022). Without question, some patients and their families will request clear direction from health professionals; when this desire is explicit, Beauchamp and Childress (2019) argue this also adheres to respect for autonomy. In acknowledgment of the reliance of patients and families on clinicians' knowledge and judgment, some authors prefer the term "collaborative decision making" to shared decision making (Clark et al., 2021).

It is typical that patients and families are overwhelmed by new information and are asked to consider highly unfamiliar concepts. For example, most people have thought very little about whether they would want tube feeding or to use a high-tech augmentative or alternative communication (AAC) device. In some circumstances, clinicians can support patient and family education through the use of decision aids. Decision aids are standardized, evidence-based tools that present information in patient-friendly terms. One example is a tool designed to help surrogate decision makers with decisions about percutaneous endoscopic gastrostomy (PEG) feeding tube placement (Mitchell et al., 2001). An inventory of decision aids is maintained by the Ottawa Hospital Research Institute (2022), the National Institute for Health Care and Excellence (NICE) in the United Kingdom

(2018), and other groups. Where such tools are available, they can serve as a helpful source of information for patients and caregivers and provide a self-paced way to review new information. Formal tools are not available for all situations and are not required to achieve shared decision making. Some examples of decision aids created to support patients with cognitive and communication impairments are provided in Appendix B.

Shared Decision Making in the Practice of Speech-Language Pathology

Shared decision making can and should be incorporated in every clinical interaction. To achieve shared decision making, the SLP listens deeply to establish what the patient and relevant caregivers understand, their concerns, values, preferences, and goals. Patient and family education includes clear, jargon-free explanations of each step of a proposed assessment or intervention together with opportunities to discuss and address questions from the

patient or their family members prior to initiating service delivery (Anderson et al., 2019). When clinicians begin a clinical relationship with genuine humility and curiosity, set aside any personal agenda or assumptions, and are prepared to change course as the patient and those closest to the patient express their understanding and goals, the SLP can build a meaningful, individualized plan for patient education, assessment, and treatment that aligns with the patient and family needs (see, for example, Sprik & Gentile, 2020).

Fortunately for the SLP in the case of Mrs. Kazem (see box below), the patient's family is aware of her strong preference and informs the SLP. This does not mean the SLP should avoid discussion of tube feeding, but this *a priori* knowledge may inform the conduct of the assessment. For example, the SLP may add steps to the assessment to identify the safest possible option for continued oral intake and conduct a more thorough assessment of associated risks. With knowledge of the likelihood that a recommendation for tube feeding will be summarily rejected, the SLP is better positioned

---

Case Example

Yasmin Kazem is 79 years old and is an inpatient in acute care after she sustained a left hemisphere cerebrovascular bleed (stroke) 3 days ago. Mrs. Kazem is referred for a clinical assessment of swallowing. The SLP completes a review of the medical record and enters the patient's room to find the patient asleep. The patient's niece is at the bedside and asks about the purpose of the assessment. Mrs. Kazem's niece responds quickly and clearly, "You do realize that she has an advance directive that states 'no feeding tube' so whatever you do, a feeding tube is not an option." The SLP learns from the patient's niece that Mrs. Kazem lost her husband 2 years ago who died hours after a feeding tube was surgically placed. Although he had been very ill and the family had delayed the decision about a feeding tube, Mrs. Kazem was convinced that the surgery hastened his death and routinely reminded all members of her family that she never wants a feeding tube. The SLP wakes the patient and finds that Mrs. Kazem is unable to restate her wishes but shakes her head vigorously "no" in agreement with her niece when asked if she would be willing to consider a feeding tube, even temporarily.

to present all recommendations with thought, care, and acknowledgment of Mrs. Kazem's previously stated wishes. Even with this information, the SLP has a duty to provide all clinical recommendations and the risks and benefits of each available option. Although the family may reject tube feeding, sometimes in the face of full information patients or family members may change their preferences based on clinical status, data, and the difference between short-term use of nonoral feeding approaches to aid rehabilitation and long-term use likely to prolong the dying process.

Prior to meeting with the patient, the SLP should conduct a thorough review of the medical record to gather information about the patient's medical status, documented discussions of wishes and goals, patient and family knowledge, understanding, and acceptance of their current status. It is important to note that patients' preferences evolve over time and as their health status changes, so even if preferences have been documented from previous discussions, flexibility and understanding of the patient's current status is critical. SLPs also benefit from conversation(s) with other members of the hospice or palliative care team who have completed their assessments or have recently seen the patient. With or without detailed information about the patient's status, the SLP should initiate an assessment with open-ended questions to assess the patient's understanding and current point of view.

Evaluations, treatments, and care plans require a clear sense of the patient's clinical status, understanding of their condition, goals, and experience with swallowing and/ or communication difficulty. From the start, the SLP should build strong rapport and aim to gain a clear sense of the patient's and caregiver's current understanding of prognosis and diagnosis. Are they realistic about their health status and likely decline? If not, do they lack information or do they prefer not to discuss an impending decline?

> **General Open-Ended Questions to Gauge Patient Perspective About Their Health Status**
>
> - Could you tell me a little about your illness and how things have changed for you more recently?
> - I'm a speech-language pathologist, or speech therapist. How have you worked with a speech therapist in the past?
> - What changes have you noticed in the way you [talk, communicate, eat or drink]?

If the SLP knows a recommendation for tube feeding is contraindicated based on a patient's advanced dementia, but the family has expressed concern about the patient's intake, it is essential to establish the family's expectations and goals before initiating an evaluation of eating, drinking, or swallowing. In this way appropriate and supportive caregiver education is embedded throughout the process of the clinical assessment and discussion of recommendations.

In practice, the SLP should invite the patient and family to participate in decision making from the beginning of each consult. The purpose of the visit should be stated at the start of the interaction with an immediate invitation to collaborate in decision making. For example, "I was asked to come and check on how you're doing with your eating and swallowing. Before we get started with that, I'd like to learn more about what you notice about your eating and drinking so I can best help you." Early on in the relationship it can be helpful to ask, "What is the best way for you to receive information?" If the patient, family, and SLP establish a pattern of shared decision making from the outset, timely and appropriate service delivery is supported and shared decision making is normalized.

Sample Questions to Establish Patient Awareness and to Convey a Goal of Shared Decision Making Before a Clinical Assessment of Swallowing

- Would you tell me what you've noticed when you eat and drink?
- Can you tell me how much effort it takes to eat or drink?
- Are there certain foods that you notice are easier for you to eat?
- How does [water, coffee, milkshake] go down for you? How about foods you have to chew?
- Are there any foods or food textures you really don't like?
- Is there anything you'd really like to be able to eat or drink?

INFORMED CONSENT IN CLINICAL CARE

In clinical care, informed consent is a voluntary agreement given by the patient as an outcome of shared decision making (Berg et al., 2001; Childress & Childress, 2020). To give informed consent, patients must understand their health status, the options available, and the risks and benefits of each alternative. When patients are active participants in each step of the purpose, methods, and potential outcomes of an assessment and integrate their personal goals and desired outcomes in treatment planning, they are best prepared to give meaningful consent for assessment or intervention. Informed consent is an outcome of an ongoing process, not a singular event. Therefore, it is important to note that patients may revoke their agreement at any time.

Legal and Ethical Requirements for Consent

The right for patients to consent to medical intervention has a long history. In the United States, the requirement to obtain permission from the patient is documented in a legal decision in which Justice Cardozo wrote, "Every human being of adult years and sound mind has a right to determine what shall be done with his own body; and a surgeon who performs an operation without his patient's consent commits an assault, for which he is liable in damages, except in cases of emergency, where the patient is unconscious, and where it is necessary to operate before consent can be obtained" (Schloendorff v. Society of New York Hospital, 1914). Although this legal case was decided in 1914, the term *informed* consent is ascribed to the legal case Salgo v. Leland Stanford, Jr. University Board of Trustees in 1957. Informed consent is also firmly established as an essential component of participation in research involving adults or children worldwide and was codified in 1947 in the Nuremberg Code (Shuster, 1997), the Declaration of Helsinki (World Medical Association, 1964), and the Belmont Report in the United States (Office for Human Research Protections, 1979). Although well established in the law, a patient's right to informed consent was not documented in professional codes of ethics that guide clinical care until considerably later and was included by the American Medical Association (AMA) in 1981 and by the American Speech-Language-Hearing Association (ASHA) in 2016 (AMA, 2013; ASHA, 2016).

Barriers to Informed Consent

True informed consent requires thoughtful and effective management of several barriers that patients and/or surrogate decision makers face in health care and other settings. Patients and families often appear to agree to assessment or intervention without full understanding for several reasons, including overreliance on written consent forms, overuse of clinical jargon, and factors that impact patient communication or cognition.

Overreliance on Written Consent Forms

Clinicians and researchers often rely on written consent forms as evidence of informed consent. However, it is widely recognized that many people sign paperwork they have not read or do not fully understand. Studies have found that grasp of consent processes and consent forms is poor among patient groups (Sherlock & Brownie, 2014), parents (Pianosi et al., 2016), and undergraduate students participating in research (Pedersen et al., 2011).

Many of us click "agree" to initiate software updates or downloads without reading or understanding the accompanying agreement. Similarly, adults in health care settings routinely sign agreements indicating they have received and understand documents even though they have not. A common example is the requirement for new patients to acknowledge receipt of privacy and/or other clinic policies as they check in for their appointment. At times, signatures are requested although policies have not been discussed or even provided for review. From the patient's perspective, the signature is a requirement to check in and start the appointment. The perceived pressure to sign is substantial, even when the individual requesting the signature is not a health professional. Pressure to sign is even greater when the power difference between professional and patient is considered.

Perception That the Goal of Consent Is to Reduce Liability Risk

When informed consent is viewed primarily as a tool to limit liability risk, this increases the likelihood that clinicians will focus on obtaining a signature rather than ensuring the components of consent have been met (Lantos, 1993). This view is captured in the shorthand phrase "I'll consent the patient," which conveys consent as something done to the patient rather than something the patient grants to the clinician (Childress & Childress, 2020). Consent forms themselves can contribute to this perception because the content is often loaded with legal and technical jargon that pose barriers for all patients (Childress & Childress, 2020). Reliance on complex, written communication is a substantial barrier for patients with limited language or literacy skills and for people with cognitive or language-based communication disorders.

The consent process is improved when clinicians and patients view consent as part of the process of patient education. Patients may require repeated explanations of risks, benefits, and options available to them, and studies support the use of interactive materials, multimedia, and materials written in clear, jargon-free language (Sherlock & Brownie, 2014).

Overuse of Clinical/Medical Jargon

Clinical professionals tend to rely heavily on technical jargon and clinical terms to communicate with one another and with patients. Medical terms are often unfamiliar to patients and families, but it can be intimidating to ask clinicians for clarification as they rattle off diagnoses, assessment tools, treatment options, or names of medications. For patients and families to achieve informed, shared decision making, it is essential for clinicians to limit the use of jargon in both written and verbal interactions.

As specialists in language and communication, SLPs hold particular awareness of language barriers. SLPs can help to identify gaps in understanding for patients and families and ensure medical terms are explained with clear, simple vocabulary.

Imbalance of Power in Clinical Relationships

When a clinician provides a patient a form and a pen, the patient will nearly always sign it, even if they do not understand what the form says. Similarly, patients may appear to agree with a plan of care that is presented verbally, even though they do not adequately understand or may not agree with the proposed plan. When a patient appears to give consent but does not fully understand or truly agree with the proposed course of action, they are less likely to follow through; this increases the risk of the patient being labelled "noncompliant."

Patients agree without adequate information for a variety of reasons. There is a fundamental difference in power in the clinician–patient relationship. Patients may be driven to please (or not disappoint) a clinician who will deliver their care. Patients rely on clinicians' expertise and often hold a reasonable belief that professionals will act to promote the patient's interests and well-being. This implicit trust in professionals who hold a position of authority is held across professional groups such as teachers, dentists, lawyers, and others. All professionals, including health workers, have an obligation to uphold the interests of the people they serve (Beauchamp & Childress, 2019). This obligation is called a fiduciary duty. Although implicit trust is often placed in health professionals, a deeper level of trust is achieved over time through shared decision making.

Patient Factors That Are Barriers to Consent

Patients with new medical diagnoses often report a period of shock, disbelief, and confusion after receiving difficult news (Jonsen et al., 2022). It is typical for patients not to recall anything about the conversation in the immediate aftermath of hearing "cancer," "Parkinson's," "terminal," or any other serious diagnostic news. Although the clinician may provide lengthy, clear explanations of implications or next steps that might be understood easily under other circumstances, this information will need to be repeated when the patient has had time to process difficult news. Patients should not be expected to make meaningful, informed decisions within hours of learning they have a life-limiting condition or terminal diagnosis.

Patients may experience other intrinsic barriers that clinicians should consider before accepting consent from a patient. Clinicians should assess whether language barriers, absence of professional interpreters or reliance

---

Barriers to Informed Consent

- Clinician overreliance on consent forms
- Clinician misconception that consent serves the purpose of legal defense
- Clinician use of medical jargon
- Power imbalance between patient and health professionals
- Patient has insufficient information
- Patient and family language barrier
- Lack of professional interpreter
- Insufficient time given for patient to process information and decide
- Patient has one or more communication disorders
- Patient has an underlying cognitive disorder
- Patient sedation or other medication-induced cognitive impairment

on family members as interpreters, illiteracy, low health literacy, disorders of language or cognition, or short-term impairments associated with medication or sedation interfere with comprehension, cognition, or expression requirements of informed decision making.

Best Practice to Obtain Informed Consent

To help patients and families achieve a clear understanding of the issues and options available, clinicians must spend time explaining the patient's status. Clinicians should avoid the use of clinical jargon. Interdisciplinary teams can facilitate patient and family education with explicit agreements within the team. For example, the team could agree on use of terminology across members of the care team to avoid confusion. For example, Zahuranec and colleagues (2018) found that patients' surrogates were confused when team members used different terms such as "stroke," "brain bleed," or "intracranial hemorrhage" to explain a cerebrovascular accident (CVA). In any setting, clinicians may need to take time to teach patients the alternate names for conditions that they may hear or that will appear in clinical records.

Informed consent is a *process* that occurs over time and is achieved when the individual has received and understands the clinical situation, the options available, and the risks and benefits of each option and then voluntarily expresses a choice. The option to forgo a given assessment or treatment should always be recognized as an option. Even when a patient signs a consent form, the scope and outcome of the conversation between clinician and patient that led to consent should be included in clinical notes.

To meet the requirements of informed consent, clinicians are obligated to ensure the patient is given:

- information about their condition in clear, understandable language free of medical jargon;
- information about the options available and the risks and benefits of each option in clear, easy-to-understand language;
- meaningful opportunities to ask questions and clear answers to those questions;
- time to consider their options, consult with others, and make a thoughtful decision that is not unduly influenced by the clinician or care team; and
- opportunities to revisit, review information, and verify understanding (e.g., teach-back) with the patient or the decision maker.

SLPs are well acquainted with assessment of comprehension and can play a key role in assisting medical teams to support comprehension, particularly for patients with language barriers and communication or cognitive disorders. One method to verify comprehension is to request that the patient or family member teach back the information requested. Clinicians often worry that a teach-back task will be insulting, but this can be overcome if the SLP establishes that the goal is to ensure understanding. Teach-back by demonstration can be incorporated naturally with "how about you give this a try" when teaching a new skill such as oral care or loading new vocabulary items on a communication board. If teach-back is based on information, one mechanism is to ask the patient or family member to practice delivery of the information to someone who is not present. For example, "We've covered a lot of information today. I know your daughter will want an update. Before you leave, let's review the main points together. How about you tell me about the (findings, next steps, procedure) as if I'm your daughter?"

Best Practices for Informed Consent

- Conduct the process of consent at *every* step of *every* clinical pathway

- Avoid the use of clinical, medical jargon

- Recognize that informed consent is a continuing process and not a single event

- Evaluate capacity to consent (decision-making capacity) as part of the consent process

- Use the teach-back (or similar) technique to confirm understanding

- Modify communication to enhance understanding

- Use professional interpreters

- Document all discussions related to decision making in the medical record; include patients' questions and clinician responses in the documentation

- Complete all discussion about risks, benefits, and options and reach voluntary agreement before presenting a consent form

- Review the consent form with the patient, give the patient (and family) time to read the consent form, and then provide a pen after the patient's questions are resolved

- Provide a copy of the consent form for the patient (and/or caregiver) to keep

- When obtaining consent for clinical research, engage someone other than the clinician to conduct the consent process to separate clinical work from research and minimize therapeutic misconception

Appropriate Use of Consent Forms

Written consent should always occur after the decision has been reached through discussion and with time to consider each option. Consent forms are routinely used for significant medical decisions, such as surgery and other invasive procedures. Consent forms are required nearly universally when patients or other volunteers agree to participate in research involving human subjects. When the process of consent is executed properly, the consent form is one last clarification of agreement that includes review of the contents of

Best Practices for Completion of Consent Forms

- Present the consent form after discussion of recommendations, alternatives, opportunities for questions, and voluntary agreement is reached

- Present the form and explain that you will not request a signature until the patient has reviewed the document with you

- Review the full written document with the patient and appropriate family caregiver(s)

- Allow reasonable time without talking for the patient or caregiver to read the entire form at their own pace

- Offer a pen for signature after joint review and time to read the form are provided

the form, time to read the form, time to ask questions, and a clear indication that signing the form is voluntary.

Procedures Conducted Without Written Consent

In clinical practice, it is routine to conduct assessments or interventions with verbal agreement rather than signed consent forms. For example, when an SLP is invited to evaluate speech, language, cognition, or swallowing in an acute care setting, it is typical to receive a medical order, review the medical record, and arrive in the patient's room to conduct an assessment. Written consent is not necessarily required in this context. However, before formal assessment takes place, the patient and family members should receive an explanation about the purpose of the visit and agree to proceed. Throughout this process, the SLP monitors for problems with the patient's speech intelligibility, cognitive function, and capacity to understand spoken language and generate verbal or gestural responses.

INFORMED REFUSAL

Patients do not always decide to follow clinical recommendations and may refuse a proposed evaluation or intervention. A refusal based on the individual's understanding of risks, benefits, and alternatives is called "informed refusal" and should be considered an equally valid outcome as informed consent (Beauchamp & Childress, 2019; Jonsen et al., 2022).

In practice, informed refusal sometimes heightens clinician concern about patient safety or raises questions about the patient's capacity to give consent because the refusal typically represents a decision by the patient that differs from the clinician's or health care team's recommendation (Jonsen et al., 2022).

On the surface, this heightened scrutiny of a patient's capacity raises reasonable questions about why clinicians readily accept patients' consent when the decision aligns with the clinician's recommendation. Capacity to consent should be confirmed as part of every consent process. However, when a patient does not agree with a proposed assessment or plan of treatment, it is appropriate to take further steps to ensure the patient's decision is fully informed and that the patient demonstrates full understanding of the risks of their decision. One such measure is the "sliding-scale criterion" (Jonsen et al., 2022). A verification of capacity after a refusal should be conducted with care and respect, usually with focus on the patient's rationale for the choice they made. With verification that the components of capacity are met, a patient's informed refusal should be honored.

In clinical settings, refusal of recommendations is too often considered "noncompliance." Noncompliance is a term that should rarely be used and differs from informed refusal in several critical ways. In a clinical context, the term "compliance" by definition implies that the patient has bent or fit their actions to the will or recommendation of the clinician. When a patient does not "comply" with recommendations, such as dysphagia precautions, use of hearing aids, or implementation of a communication device, rather than characterizing the patient's actions as an act of noncompliance, it is worthwhile to revisit the patient's goals, explore patient-perceived barriers, and reevaluate the recommendation in partnership with the patient.

It is problematic to consider a patient's refusal of intervention a wish to die or to hasten death (American Academy of Pediatrics [AAP], 2000; Jonsen et al., 2022). For example, refusal of tube feeding from the patient's perspective may reflect a preference to eat and drink or to socialize during meals rather than a wish to die. Similarly, when an infant, child, or adult who is not alert or aware removes a tube, it is most likely that the tube is causing discomfort or pain that should be assessed and treated rather than interpreting the patient's action is indicative of an intent to hasten death.

Clinicians who work with patients at EoL should ensure the use of clear terminology in all interactions with members of the health care team, patients, and families related to withholding (never starting intervention), withdrawing (stopping intervention), assisted suicide, and euthanasia. These terms hold distinct meaning in bioethics and in the law. It is not uncommon for family members to use incorrect terms such as "suicide" when a patient refuses life-sustaining treatment, such as ventilation, dialysis, or tube feeding. These terms, together with ethical and legal considerations, are summarized in Table 3–1.

ASSESSMENT OF A PATIENT'S CAPACITY TO DECIDE

A core role for clinicians throughout the process of shared decision making is to assess each patient's capacity to give informed consent or informed refusal. The term "competence" is often used incorrectly in this context, so it is important to differentiate the term *competence* from *decision-making capacity* because they have very different implications and applications in clinical care.

Distinction Between Competence and Decision-Making Capacity

Competence is a legal term, while decision-making capacity (DMC) is a clinical construct (Beauchamp & Childress, 2019; Lo, 2020). In the United States and in many other countries, legal competency is automatic when one

becomes a legal adult. In the United States, competence to consent to medical treatment is granted at age 18, along with a host of other legal rights and responsibilities, including the right to vote, consent to marriage, open a bank account, or enlist in the military. In some jurisdictions there may be slight variations in the law that specify a different age requirement for any given right or responsibility. Because legal competence is assumed for adults, competence can only be restricted or removed through legal proceedings.

Legal competency determinations are somewhat routine for young adults with developmental cognitive disorders and typically occur before age 18 to ensure continuity of decision-making authority. Some families may elect to pursue guardianship through the courts when a family member has no expectation of recovery; for example, as cognitive decline progresses with dementia. However, among other clinical populations, legal competency proceedings are uncommon. For example, it is rare for families to seek court intervention after an acute event such as a stroke, traumatic injury, or altered cognitive status associated with new metastases to the brain. Consequently, in the majority of clinical cases, DMC is determined by clinicians rather than through the court system.

Assessment of DMC is conducted for each clinical decision and, unlike legal competence, DMC is not all encompassing. It is recognized that DMC can fluctuate over time, even within a single day. For example, patients who require pain medication may temporarily lose capacity due to sedative effects of medication or in the minutes or hours after receiving unexpected bad news. Capacity is also assessed in a context of the weight of the decision at hand, referred to as a "sliding scale." Thus, a person may have capacity to make one decision, but lack the capacity for a different decision. For example, a patient with dementia might be able to consider the risks and

Table 3–1. Terminology Differentiating Ethical and Legal Considerations Associated With Withholding or Withdrawing Treatment, Assisted Death, and Euthanasia

Action	Allowing the Patient to Die		Hastening Death	
	Withhold Life-Sustaining Treatment	Withdraw Life-Sustaining Treatment	Assisted Suicide*	Voluntary Euthanasia*
Example	Intervention such as tube feeding is not started based on an informed decision by patient or surrogate or advance directive	Intervention such as ventilation is stopped based on an informed decision by patient or surrogate or advance directive	Patient who qualifies under specific criteria is given a prescription for medications they can self-administer to end their own life	Physician, nurse practitioner, or other health professional administers medication with the intent of ending the patient's life
Legal Considerations in the United States	Permissible. Withholding and withdrawing life-sustaining treatment are considered morally, ethically, and legally equivalent (President's Commission, 1983; Macauley, 2018).		Permissible by statute in California, Colorado, Hawaii, Maine, New Jersey, New Mexico, Oregon, Vermont, Washington, and Washington DC (Roehr, 2021)	Not permitted in the United States
Legal Considerations Around the World	Permissible in most jurisdictions. Withholding and withdrawing life-sustaining treatment are generally considered morally, ethically, and legally equivalent (Macauley, 2018; Vincent, 2005).		Permissible in some states and territories in Australia, Belgium, Canada, Netherlands, Spain, and Switzerland, with legislation pending in other countries (Roehr, 2021)	Permissible in some countries for example, Belgium, Canada, Columbia, and the Netherlands (Roehr, 2021)

*The term "euthanasia" is often qualified "voluntary" to specify euthanasia at the request of the patient and "involuntary" administration without patient consent (Beauchamp & Childress, 2019; Jonsen et al., 2022; Vincent, 2005). Canada adopted the term "Medical Assistance in Dying" (MAiD), which incorporates both assisted suicide and voluntary euthanasia (Bill C-14, 2016). Specific legislation is subject to change. Clinicians should verify ethical and legal standards where they practice and over time.

benefits of adjusting pain medication, but not able to consider all the risks and benefits of a foot amputation. Because DMC fluctuates and is assessed for each specific decision using a sliding scale, a patient's capacity to decide is assessed separately for every clinical decision (Appelbaum & Grisso, 1988; Lo, 2020; Sachs, 2000). Capacity is evaluated specifically for the decision in question and not through use of general clinical tools such as the Mini-Mental Status Exam (MMSE; Sachs, 2000). Members of the clinical team may consult with the courts in competency rulings, but generally, DMC is usually evaluated clinically while competence is evaluated through the legal system (Appelbaum & Grisso, 1988; Beauchamp & Childress, 2019).

Components of Decision-Making Capacity

DMC requires a patient to demonstrate that they understand their health situation, the options available, and the risks and benefits of each option. Next, the patient must demonstrate the cognitive reasoning skills required to weigh the risks and benefits to reach a rational decision and then express their decision definitively (Appelbaum & Grisso, 1988).

It is important to note that *reasoning and rationality* does not mean the patient must make the decision the clinician might make in this circumstance; rather, the patient is asked to explain how they arrived at their decision. The logic the patient has used to make their

---

Case Example

Mr. Facundo is a 76-year-old patient who recently sustained a cerebellar bleed and is transferred to inpatient rehabilitation after 10 days of acute care. Dysphagia precautions are in place and, on a reevaluation of swallowing function, aspiration on all food consistencies and liquids is noted. Mr. Facundo definitively states he wants to eat and drink and will not consider alternative approaches to nutrition and hydration support. Immediately, a member of the team questions whether he has the capacity to make this decision so soon after a stroke.

An ethics consultation is requested and the clinical ethics team talks with Mr. Facundo about his medical status. They ask Mr. Facundo why he will not consider the possibility of tube feeding. Mr. Facundo states, "I understand that some of my food or water will probably go to my lungs and that might make me cough or I could get pneumonia. I know if I get sick

I might have to go back to the hospital. But the thing is, I've been eating food and drinking water and coffee since my stroke two weeks ago and I'm doing ok. If I start having problems, I'll rethink the tube, but for now, I'd rather keep eating."

Although the SLP and other members of the team might doubt they would make this choice for themselves, Mr. Facundo's response demonstrates (a) understanding of the problem, (b) understanding of the options available, (c) understanding of the risks of the decision he's making, (d) a rational explanation for his decision, and (e) a clearly expressed choice. Mr. Facundo has met all the criteria for DMC and his informed decision about continued oral intake should be honored. Recommendations for strategies to support the safest possible intake, monitoring for signs of pneumonia or complications, and Mr. Facundo's preferences in the event of complications should be established.

Components of Decision-Making Capacity (DMC)

- Understands the current health-related situation
- Understands relevant information including options available and the risks and benefits of each option
- Demonstrates reasoning and rationality
- Expresses a choice

(Appelbaum & Grisso, 1988; Grisso & Appelbaum, 1998)

decision should be clear. Clinicians may ask the patient to explain how they reached the decision and may consider whether the decision is consistent with previous decisions or discussions and/or the patient's stated values and goals (Lo, 2020).

Patients' capacity for consent can be promoted through consistent patient education and partnership in shared decision making.

Role of the Speech-Language Pathologist in Assessment of Capacity

The SLP's expertise in differentiation, identification, and management of speech, language, cognitive, and hearing disorders that impact communication can assist in overcoming assumptions made by members of the care team and patients' families. The components of DMC require that the patient demonstrate language comprehension, language expression, and cognitive reasoning. Each of these domains falls within the scope of practice for SLPs (ASHA, 2016). For many patients, but particularly for patients' communication and/

or cognitive conditions that may be barriers to demonstration of DMC, the SLP should play an essential role in the determination of DMC.

Patients with any form of communication barrier are at risk for exclusion from decisions about their care because others underestimate their DMC (Appelbaum & Grisso, 1988; Carling-Rowland & Wahl, 2017; Leskuski, 2009; Sachs, 2000). SLP consultation or intervention can be essential for patients who have a communication impairment to demonstrate DMC, particularly when communication barriers are present. Examples of ways in which an SLP can advocate for patients are provided in Table 3–2. If a patient's capacity to participate in their own health care decisions is uncertain because of limited communication or cognition, the SLP's assessment of language and cognitive function and recommendations related to communication may provide essential information for the medical care team that allows the patient to participate and to direct their own care. When patients are at risk of losing communication or cognitive skills, the SLP can encourage patients who have DMC to discuss their preferences for treatment and decision making with their loved ones and the care team to clarify their wishes in the event they lose DMC.

Patients with communication impairments are also at risk of others overestimating their capacity. For example, a patient with aphasia who readily agrees to statements and questions with a stereotypic utterance such as "yep" may appear to understand a physician, family member, or other health professional better than they really do. This tendency to appear agreeable can produce a false appearance of comprehension, which can lead to an assumption that the patient has given consent. It is crucial to clarify what the patient does and does not understand to ensure the patient has the capacity to give consent.

Table 3–2. Examples of Strategies for Speech-Language Pathologists to Support Participation in Decision Making for Patients With Communication Barriers

All patients across settings	• Eliminate use of medical and professional jargon • Reduce background noise when possible (e.g., turn off the TV) • Ensure speaker's face is well lit • Supplement verbal information with written information
Patient whose primary language differs from provider's	• Use a professional interpreter • Ensure consent forms are available in the appropriate language • Do not ask a patient to sign a form they cannot read
Patient with low vision or low literacy	• Review all written materials thoroughly and document the review • Identify audio alternatives such as text-to-speech reader • Do not rely on written materials for patient education; consider audio- and/or video-based instruction • Do not ask a patient to sign a form they cannot read; document consent discussions in clinical notes
Patient with hearing impairment	• Review audiology and hearing health–related records • Ensure access to functioning hearing aids, cochlear implant, and/or assistive technologies • Teach bedside or home visiting nurse and other members of the care team how to complete a hearing aid check • Teach caregivers and health team members essential strategies such as speak clearly, preserve visual cues, allow time for patient to identify the speaker in group conversations
Patient with tracheotomy	• Implement use of speaking valve (e.g., Passy-Muir) if tolerated by patient • Provide access to appropriate communication board or device and support routine use if speaking valve not tolerated or as alternative
Patient with limited capacity for speech or language production	• Verify accuracy of comprehension via yes/no responses (e.g., point, eye gaze, hand squeeze, blink) • Teach care team members and family how to ask effective yes/no questions • Provide access to appropriate communication board or device and support routine use
Patient with weak or limited voice production	• Implement voice amplification • Ensure communication partners have adequate hearing
Patient with intact comprehension at sentence level	• Coach members of the health care team to provide information in small chunks and free of jargon, and to eliminate extraneous sidebar comments
Patient who benefits from multimodal communication	• Identify strategies that maximize comprehension (e.g., written or pictorial cues) • Support implementation of modified patient education and consent documents
Patient with memory or other cognitive deficits	• Ask the patient who they would like to have with them when clinical teaching or instructions are provided • Supplement verbal information with written summary • Use teach-back to verify understanding

When the Patient Does Not Have Decision-Making Capacity

When a patient is unable to participate in decision making, it is essential to determine whether the lack of capacity is temporary (e.g., patient is sedated or recovering from general anesthesia) or long term (e.g., irreversible cognitive impairment). When feasible, direct communication with the patient about treatment decisions is strongly preferred over decisions made by the patient's surrogate decision maker. Studies of patient–surrogate pairs find that surrogates' estimations of their loved one's preferences are inaccurate about one-third of the time, with some studies showing a level of agreement that would be expected by chance (Shalowitz et al., 2006; Smuker et al., 2000; Spalding, 2021). Therefore, if a patient's loss of DMC is known to be temporary or there is strong potential to restore DMC, any decisions that can be postponed should wait until the patient is able to participate.

If the patient's capacity to make a particular decision is not clear, the team may call for a psychiatric or neuropsychological consult to determine whether the patient has DMC. These professions are historically connected with legal determination of competency, particularly for patients with mental health conditions. However, for patients with communication barriers or disorders, the SLP can play an essential role as a consultant to the care team or in the context of a DMC determination. If adaptation of communication strategies is needed for the patient to demonstrate DMC, the SLP should guide this process. Specific interventions to facilitate comprehension and/or expression are discussed in Chapter 4 and in the literature based on the patient's specific communication needs. For example, patients with aphasia may initially appear to have inadequate capacity, but may be able to participate and give informed consent with modifications to communication (Carling-

Rowland & Wahl, 2017; Jayes & Palmer, 2014; Stein & Brady Wagner, 2006)

If a patient is unlikely to regain DMC or if decisions must be made while the patient temporarily lacks DMC, the team should follow a process that includes review of any advance care planning documents the patient may have executed, such as written advance directives (such as a living will), advance medical orders, and/or a previously identified surrogate decision maker.

ADVANCE CARE PLANNING

Establishing goals of care and advance care planning are core components of hospice and palliative care (see Chapter 1). Advance care planning encompasses a broad range of mechanisms through which patients can express their preferences. Advance care plans allow patients to establish medical orders with their physician, convey directives and goals in the event that they lose DMC or are otherwise unable to convey their wishes, and/or identify someone to make decisions on their behalf. Advance care plans are particularly helpful when executed in a context of a known diagnosis and health trajectory or when patients want to identify a particular individual to act on their behalf if they lose DMC.

Advance Medical Orders

In the United States, the nationally recognized Transportable Physician Orders for Patient Preferences (TPOPP) or Portable Medical Order Form (known as POLST) is a specific subtype of a health directive designed to be completed by persons with serious illness or medical frailty (Center for Practical Bioethics, 2022; National POLST, 2022). POLST forms are completed by the patient in conjunction with their physician and become standing medical orders that travel with the patient across settings.

Advance medical orders (e.g., POLST) allow patients to indicate their preferences for EoL interventions such as cardiopulmonary resuscitation (CPR), tube feeding, use of intravenous fluids or medication, and use of mechanical ventilation. These documents, if signed by the patient and their primary physician or in health care settings, yield "do not resuscitate," "do not intubate," and other medical orders that are entered into the medical record.

Advance Directives

Written health directives are statements of preferences related to medical interventions that can be completed by any adult (National Institute on Aging, 2022). For example, an adult may determine that they do *not* want a feeding tube to prolong the dying process and can complete a living will to notify both professionals and family members of this preference.

The Living Will

Healthy adults are able to complete living wills or similar advance directive documents to detail their preferences for health interventions in the event that the person loses DMC and is terminally or irreversibly ill. While these documents can be helpful to guide medical decision making, they are subject to interpretation at the time of implementation, particularly if considerable time has lapsed between completion of the document(s) and when medical decisions are made. While it is strongly encouraged that individuals review and revise their directives annually, many people do not revisit their advance directives. Individuals' family and life circumstances, values, and lived experiences may change considerably between the time of completion of the living will and when they are applied, which in some cases will call into question whether the individual would want their previous wishes upheld.

The case of Ms. Naidoo (see box below) illustrates the difficulty of anticipating in advance directives every possible decision that might need to be made during the dying pro-

---

Case Example

Thembi Naidoo is a 67-year-old woman with recurrent breast cancer. The cancer metastasized and Ms. Naidoo opted to forgo any further cancer intervention. She stated a preference to live her life. She lives alone and takes care of her daily needs, enjoys gardening, and gets together with friends several times a week. Ms. Naidoo completed advance directive documents including a living will that states she does not want her life prolonged using a ventilator, feeding tubes, or other life support. Although it is not certain what her life expectancy is, her physicians are confident that given her general health, she could expect to live for another year. A few weeks after completing her advance care plan, Ms. Naidoo developed community-acquired pneumonia and was hospitalized. Ms. Naidoo was quite ill with high fever and was unable to make decisions for herself. The care team recommended brief use of a ventilator to support her breathing, but they are uncertain about how to interpret her living will in the context of an acute but likely reversible health issue.

cess. Ms. Naidoo was not imminently dying, but did have a written advance directive stating she did not want to use ventilator support to prolong the dying process. Fortunately, Ms. Naidoo also completed a durable power of attorney for health care form and named her daughter as her surrogate decision maker. The patient's daughter was confident that this short-term use of a ventilator for a reversible condition was not what her mother contemplated when she completed the living will.

Identify a Surrogate (or Substitute) Decision Maker

When patients are unable to make decisions for themselves, someone other than the health care team is identified and is empowered to act on behalf of the patient. Many countries and jurisdictions allow adults to identify someone they would like to make decisions on their behalf through the process of advance care planning.

Optimally, adult patients will have named a surrogate decision maker to act on their behalf and will have also discussed their wishes with that person. It is estimated that approximately one-third of adults in the United States have completed an advance directive (Yadav et al., 2017). The documentation required to name a surrogate decision maker varies with respect to whether one or more witnesses are required, who may serve as a witness, and whether the person named must acknowledge their role in writing. It is important to note that these surrogate decision makers are only empowered to act when the person lacks the capacity to make their own decisions.

There is considerable variation in terminology used for the role of a decision maker empowered to act on behalf of an adult patient. Some terms have specific legal meaning; for example, the term "guardian" is used frequently. However, very few patients have a

formal guardian appointed through the court system. Parents who make decisions for their children who are under the age of 18 are also referred to as legal guardians. Adults with significant developmental cognitive disorders are likely to have a legal guardian. However, guardianship is rare for adults because after acute events such as stroke or brain injury there is a clinical expectation of recovery, so very few families initiate complex and potentially costly legal proceedings to appoint a guardian. In most cases, a surrogate or proxy decision maker is identified. For the purpose of this chapter, "surrogate decision maker" is the primary term used. Alternate terms used in clinical settings are summarized in Table 3–3.

For some patients and in any jurisdiction that does not recognize common-law, lesbian, or gay relationships, patients are well served to provide instructions about who they would like to make decisions on their behalf (Acquaviva, 2017). In the absence of a written directive that names a surrogate decision maker, patients can be asked to identify who they would like to make decisions for them if they lose the capacity to decide. Any such verbally (or otherwise) communicated directive should be documented in the medical record.

Who Serves as a Surrogate Decision Maker When the Patient's Wishes Are Not Known? If the individual does not have a plan of care and a surrogate decision maker has not been identified, then legal statutory guidance can be used to identify who should be authorized to decide on behalf of the patient. In the United States, the Uniform Health-Care Decisions Act (1994) specifies the hierarchy of persons who may act on behalf of the patient with the caveat that any selected person must be "reasonably available." The hierarchy of authority to serve as a surrogate decision maker when there is no

Table 3–3. Terms Used in Health Care Settings and the Literature to Identify the Person Authorized to Make Health Care Decisions on Behalf of a Patient

Role of the Decision Maker	Terms Used
Decision maker(s) for a child	• Parent • Guardian
Court-appointed decision maker	• Legal guardian • Conservator
Individual designated by the patient through advance care planning or advance directive	• Surrogate decision maker • Agent • Attorney-in-fact • Durable power of attorney for health care • Medical power of attorney • Health care proxy • Medical proxy • Proxy • Proxy decision maker • Surrogate
Decision maker identified by default	• Next of kin • Health care surrogate • Health care representative • Medical treatment decision maker • Proxy • Substitute decision maker • Surrogate decision maker

legal guardian *and* the patient's preference is unknown is:

1. spouse, unless legally separated;
2. adult child;
3. parent;
4. adult sibling; or
5. an adult who has exhibited special care and concern for the patient, who is familiar with the patient's personal values, and who is reasonably available

This general hierarchy does not mitigate disputes, particularly when there is more than one person in a given role such as mul-tiple adult children of the patient. However, research supports general satisfaction with the hierarchy. Cox Hayley and colleagues (1996) found that most individuals who would have chosen someone else as their surrogate were "not troubled" by discrepancies that were introduced when the hierarchy selection process was applied in a hypothetical research scenario.

Health professionals are almost never empowered to make decisions on behalf of a patient who has lost capacity for decision making. In many jurisdictions, the law specifies that employees of a health care facility may *not* make decisions on a patient's behalf unless they are a blood relative (e.g., Uniform

Health-Care Decisions Act, 1994). However, in very limited circumstances, medical teams may be empowered to make unilateral decisions about a patient's care. Crisis standards of care policies (Institute of Medicine, 2012) are an example that gained attention throughout the height of the COVID-19 pandemic.

Written advance directives must be completed by the individual. In most jurisdictions, one or more witnesses are required to verify that the form was completed by the individual at a time they were of "sound mind" and completed the form(s) without coercion.

Barriers to Advance Care Planning

Most adults are in favor of advance care planning, but relatively few people execute written directives. A 2020 scoping review found 80% to 90% of people across studies think advance care planning is important and that less than one third of adults have a written advance directive (Grant et al., 2020). Although the benefits of advance care planning seem appealing at first glance, there are several barriers that complicate advance care planning. Cultural, social, and systems barriers limit discussions about death and dying. Throughout this book, we have identified the human inclination to avoid the topic of death and dying. Clinicians, patients, and family members are all susceptible to this inclination that leads to avoidance of advance care planning. Discussions about preferences in hypothetical complex medical situations can be overwhelming. Strategies to support clinician truth telling, breaking bad news, and difficult conversations are addressed in Chapter 1 (see also Back et al., 2009).

It is a common misconception that the process is cumbersome or costly. Many people believe, incorrectly, that a lawyer is needed to execute legal advance directives. These documents are readily available online and in health care facilities in many jurisdictions.

Individuals can usually complete advance directives at home. In the United States, most states adhere to the Uniform Health-Care Decisions Act (1994), although there remain state-specific variations in implementation. Clinicians should verify, by statute, the specifics of medical decision laws in the jurisdictions where they practice.

A second misconception is a fear that beneficial intervention might be withheld because the documents exist. It is important for clinicians and patients to understand that advance directives, such as the living will, are only used when the patient loses capacity to make decisions. Similarly, it is helpful to clarify that a named surrogate decision maker only has authority to make decisions when the patient cannot decide for themselves.

Even when advance directive documents are completed, it is not possible to predict all the decisions that will need to be made in the future, even when there is a known diagnosis, such as in the case of Ms. Naidoo (above). These tools are intended to uphold the patient's autonomy even after they have lost DMC, but statements of preference that precede actual health decisions are fraught with flaws (Fagerlin & Schneider, 2004). Perhaps the most difficult barrier associated with advance care planning is that people's priorities, preferences, and perspectives change as they experience disease and disability.

Change in Perspective With Experience of Disease and Disability

People who experience new onset health changes frequently report that their perspective shifts substantially with lived experience. For example, Nancy Mairs (1996) writes about her experience of the progression of multiple sclerosis:

> Everybody, well or ill, disabled or not, imagines a boundary of suffering and loss beyond which, she or he is certain, life will no lon-

ger be worth living. I know that I do. I also know that my line, far from being scored in stone, has inched across the sands of my life: at various times, I could not possibly do without long walks on the beach or rambles through the woods; use a cane, a brace, a wheelchair; stop teaching; give up driving; let someone else put on and take off my underwear. One at a time, with the encouragement of others, I have taken each of these (highly figurative) steps. Now I believe my limit to lie at George's death, but I am prepared to let it move if it will. When I reach the wall, I think I'll know. Meanwhile, I go on being, now more than ever, the woman I once thought I could never bear to be. (Mairs, 1996, pp. 121–122)

The observations of individuals' shift in perspective over time is widely represented in narrative literature (see Appendix C) and is consistent with research findings that show a systematic tendency of healthy persons, including health professionals, to underestimate the quality of life of individuals with disabilities (Gerhart et al., 1994; Gerhart & Corbet, 1995; Lagu et al., 2022).

In the context of life-limiting conditions, individuals who experience gradual changes in health over time can be expected to change their priorities and goals of care, even when they have made clear statements of preference in the past. Because people's preferences fluctuate over time, it is essential that patients retain the capacity to communicate decisions for as long as possible. Plans of care require ongoing, dynamic consultation with the patient about their preferences over time. This is especially true of advance wishes that were documented when the person was healthy (Elliott & Elliott, 1991; Neher, 2004).

The SLP should maintain open communication and flexibility at each step of any disease trajectory. For example, a patient may initially reject the use of AAC, but over time and with experience they may later embrace an alternate form of communication. Similarly, patients may not be able to imagine life without the pleasure of eating or drinking, but later express relief when they initiate tube feeding for delivery of medication, food, and/or fluids (Bicakli et al., 2019; Pollens et al., 2009). The reverse is also true. Patients may initially agree to tube feeding or request an alternative form of communication and later reject the intervention. Due to the likelihood of change in priorities and needs over time, an ongoing goal for the SLP is to support patients' access to communication for as long as the patient is able.

Despite these difficulties in interpretation, so few people develop written directives that when they exist, health care professionals and family members pay close attention to those preferences as a guide when the patient can no longer indicate their wishes. Ideally, the individual will have named a surrogate decision maker who can be consulted and asked to interpret what the patient would have wanted. Despite the uncertainties introduced through advance directives and the considerable burden assumed by a surrogate decision maker, the surrogate experiences less uncertainty and less guilt 1 year later if the patient's wishes are known (Wendler & Rid, 2011).

Steps to Take When No Advance Care Plan Is Available

When patients are unable to make decisions and their preferences are not known, the health care team has a more complex set of steps to take to make decisions. In most circumstances in which an urgent or emergent decision is required, neither the patient's wishes nor a surrogate decision maker is available. In such cases, decisions typically err on the side of treatment (Lo, 2020). For example, if the patient's heart stops and there are no existing do not resuscitate orders, the team will typically attempt CPR. For less urgent decisions, steps can be taken to identify an appropriate surrogate decision maker (see steps for selection above).

The Role of a Surrogate Decision Maker

The role of the surrogate decision maker is to act on behalf of the patient (sometimes labeled as "an agent" for the patient). This responsibility requires that the surrogate represent the values and preferences of the patient, not their own preferences. Ideally, a patient will have discussed their preferences, goals, and values with their surrogate and/or have left a record of their preferences in written form.

Clinicians can support the surrogate by maintaining focus on the patient's preferences and values to encourage "substituted judgement" and ask, "What do you think [your mother] would have wanted if she could tell us right now?" This question shifts surrogates away from the burden of deciding what is best, can unify family members who have differing perspectives about the "right thing" to do, and holds the patient's perspective at the center (Anderson et al., 2019; Macauley, 2018).

DECISION MAKING FOR CHILDREN AND ADOLESCENTS

Care for children with life-limiting conditions is complex and best managed through an interdisciplinary team with expertise in the specific condition and in palliative care (AAP, 2000; Linebarger et al., 2022; see also Chapter 6).

Parents routinely take children to medical appointments and give permission for assessments and interventions for medical care and rehabilitation services, including speech-language therapy. Parents are expected to know

their child best and serve as the presumptive decision makers for children in most circumstances (Buchanan & Brock, 1989; Ross, 1998). The role of parent as a decision maker is to weigh and balance the best interests of the child. This differs from the role of a surrogate for an adult with previously expressed preferences, values, and goals (Clark et al., 2021).

In all pediatric care, clinicians navigate decision making with parents and children/adolescents (Macauley, 2018), most often in the context of an interdisciplinary team. When parents must navigate EoL care for their child, it is expected that they will require ongoing support associated with decision making (AAP, 2000; Macauley, 2018; Rapoport et al., 2013).

Inclusion of Children in Decision Making

The American Academy of Pediatrics (AAP, 2016) recommends that children and adolescents "should participate in decision making commensurate with their development, they should provide assent to care whenever reasonable" (p. 1484). Assent is an agreement given by a patient who lacks full decision-making authority. In clinical contexts, a child should be aware of the name of their medical condition, what the provider plans to do, what to expect, and the reason for the assessment or intervention proposed. Some details such as costs, risks, benefits, and alternatives may be omitted based on an assessment of the individual's capacity to interpret the information (AAP, 2016). The concept of assent is also applicable to adults who lack DMC, but it is most often discussed in the pediatrics literature in the contexts of both clinical care and research.

While the AAP is focused primarily on the role of children and adolescents in medical decisions, the inclusion of children and teens in decisions about their own care is also increasingly emphasized in education settings. For example, many school systems routinely include children in Individualized Education Plan (IEP) meetings. From the age of 14 years, adolescents must be invited to attend their IEP meetings, but are not required to be present (U.S. Department of Education, 2017). While the parents give formal consent through signing IEP documents, children and adolescents are recognized as a critical part of the review of progress, goal setting, and transition planning. The inclusion of children in decision making about their own care contributes to effective transitions to adulthood, at which time the teen takes full authority for medical decision making (AAP, 2016).

In Chapter 6, Costello and Santiago discuss the need to consider a child's cognitive developmental stage rather than age with respect to understanding and integrating any child's views on illness, death, dying, and medical care. This is particularly important when working with children who have serious illness.

Although children may not have full authority to make decisions for themselves, SLPs can and should empower children as participants in their own care to the extent that the child is able.

Role of Very Young Children in Decision Making

Infants, toddlers, and preschool-aged children are fully reliant on parents (or other guardians) and caregivers for all aspects of their care. Nevertheless, even young children should be offered a brief explanation of what the clinician is doing and why. For example, when conducting an oral exam, a demonstration using yourself, a puppet, or a parent is an effective way to show a young child what you plan to do. Some children will engage with the task, such as holding the light for you while

you look in a parent's mouth. A simple explanation such as "I'd like to look in your mouth now so I can see your teeth and everything in there. Let's take a look!" is truthful and effective for many young children. Early agreement (assent) is evident when the child voluntarily opens their mouth for the clinician. It is advisable to avoid asking very young children "Do you want to . . . open your mouth?" in the form of a question which often yields a quick, unconsidered "no." Where possible, children can exert small forms of autonomy through choice questions such as "Should we play with the barn first or read a book first?" Either option should be an equally valid choice for clinical purposes. For children who are able to generate spontaneous communication, end the session with "What are your questions for me?"

Role of School-Aged Children in Decision Making

As cognitive development progresses, a child's capacity to collaborate with their parents and clinicians in decision making increases. While parents (or guardians) remain solely responsible for consent, as a child gains cognitive and communication skills, they build capacity to give informal agreement through assent. It is expected, for example, that typically developing school-aged children will be able to engage in self-assessment of their speech, reading, and language understanding and to contribute to goal setting.

Children with chronic and/or serious illness may develop specific areas of strength such as sophisticated vocabulary as they learn medical terms and the patterns of medical clinic or hospital visits. However, children with substantial health concerns may also show specific gaps in reading, language, or cognitive function. Therefore, it is essential to conduct thoughtful assessments of language and cognition in this age group (see also Chapter 6).

Role of Adolescents in Decision Making

Adolescents' language and cognitive skills are often sufficiently developed for the teen to demonstrate the components of DMC (AAP, 2016; Baltag et al., 2022; Macauley, 2018). In ideal circumstances, adolescents participate in decision making alongside their parents and health care providers (AAP, 2016).

While most jurisdictions default to the age of majority as the age at which young adults are authorized to make medical decisions, many jurisdictions recognize the role of the "mature minor," or adolescents who demonstrate DMC and have reached a specific age (e.g., 14 or 16 years of age) (Macauley, 2018). Mature minor statutes and rules may limit the type of care adolescents can seek independently and with confidentiality. Where such laws exist, teens are most often granted access to care they might not seek otherwise such as reproductive, sexual, or mental health and/or substance abuse treatment (Sigman & O'Connor, 1991). The mature minor doctrine has been invoked when adolescents want to make other medical decisions, such as forgoing chemotherapy or medical interventions (Benston, 2016).

> "The informed decision of an adolescent or young adult nearing death to refuse further life-sustaining medical treatment ought to be respected."—AAP, 2000, p. 354

The role of adolescents in health care decisions is also recognized as relevant and important in EoL decisions (AAP, 2000; Macauley, 2018). However, these decisions are exceptionally complex from ethical and legal perspectives and are best handled at an individual level by an interdisciplinary pediatric palliative care team with the expertise to navigate and support teens and their families through EoL decision making.

SUMMARY

Communication is essential for patients at every age and throughout the process of dying. A model of collaborative decision making should be established from the outset of the clinical relationship to normalize and support each patient's autonomy. To participate in shared decision making and informed consent, patients and their families require clear communication about diagnosis, prognosis, and available options (Gonella et al., 2019). SLPs have the knowledge and skills to assess patients' comprehension and cognitive function, to maximize patients' capacity for language expression, and to preserve the patient's participation in decision making for as long as possible. Capacity to decide is determined for each decision and may fluctuate for a given patient within the same day. Children and teens should participate in care decisions based on their developmental, cognitive, and language capacity. For additional resources, see Appendix C.

REFERENCES

Acquaviva, K. D. (2017). *LGBTQ-inclusive hospice and palliative care: A practical guide to transforming professional practice.* Harrington Park Press.

American Academy of Pediatrics. (2000). Palliative care for children. *Pediatrics, 106*(2), 351–357.

American Academy of Pediatrics. (2016). Informed consent in decision-making in pediatric practice. *Pediatrics, 138*(2), e1484–1491. https://doi.org/10.1542/peds.2016-1484

American Medical Association. (2013). The AMA Code of Medical Ethics' opinion on informing patients about treatment options. Opinion

8.08—Informed consent. *American Medical Association Journal of Ethics*, *15*(1), 28.

American Speech-Language-Hearing Association. (2016). *Scope of practice in speech-language pathology.* https://www.asha.org/siteassets/publications/sp2016-00343.pdf

Anderson, R. J., Bloch, S., Armstrong, M., Stone, P. C., & Low, J. T. S. (2019). Communication between healthcare professionals and relatives of patients approaching the end of life: A systematic review of qualitative evidence. *Palliative Medicine*, *33*(8), 926–941. https://doi.org/10.1177/0269216319852007

Appelbaum, P. S., & Grisso, T. (1988). Assessing patients' capacities to consent to treatment. *New England Journal of Medicine*, *319*(25), 1635–1638.

Back, A., Arnold, R., & Tulsky, J. (2009). *Mastering communication with seriously ill patients: Balancing honesty with empathy and hope.* Cambridge University Press.

Baltag, V., Takeuchi, Y., Guthold, R., & Ambresin, A.-E. (2022). Assessing and supporting adolescents' capacity for autonomous decision-making in health-care settings: New guidance from the World Health Organization. *Journal of Adolescent Health*, *71*, 10–13. https://doi.org/10.1016/j.jadohealth.2022.04.005

Beauchamp, T. L., & Childress, J. F. (2019). *Principles of biomedical ethics* (8th ed.). Oxford University Press.

Benston, S. (2016). Not of minor consequence? Medical decision-making autonomy and the mature minor doctrine. *Indiana Health Law Review*, *13*(1), 1–16. https://doi.org/10.18060/3911.0011

Berg, J. W., Appelbaum, P. S., Lidz, C. W., & Parker, L. S. (2001). *Informed consent: Legal theory and clinical practice* (2nd ed.). Oxford University Press.

Bicakli, D. H., Sari, H. Y., Yilmaz, M., Cetingul, N., & Kantar, M. (2019). Nasogastric tube feeding experiences in pediatric oncology patients and their mothers. *Gastroenterology Nursing*, *42*(3), 286–293.

Buchanan, A. E., & Brock, D. W. (1989). *Deciding for others: The ethics of surrogate decision making.* Cambridge University Press.

Carling-Rowland, A., & Wahl, J. (2017). The evaluation of capacity to make admissions decisions: Is it a fair process for individuals with communication barriers? *Medical Law International*, *19*(3), 171–190. https://doi.org/10.1177/0968533321001000301

Childress, J. F., & Childress, M. D. (2020). What does the evolution from informed consent to shared decision making teach us about authority in health care? *AMA Journal of Ethics*, *22*, E423–E429.

Center for Practical Bioethics. (2022). *Transportable physician orders for patient preferences (TPOPP).* https://www.practicalbioethics.org/programs/transportable-physician-orders-for-patient-preferences-tpopp-polst/

Clark, J. D., Lewis-Newby, M., Kon, A. A., & Morrison, W. (2021). Serious pediatric illness: A spectrum of clinician directiveness in collaborative decision making. In J. D. Lantos (Ed.), *The ethics of shared decision making.* Oxford.

Cox Hayley, D., Stern, R., Stocking, C., & Sachs, G. A. (1996). The application of health care surrogate laws to older populations: How good a match? *Journal of the American Geriatrics Society*, *44*, 185–188.

Cruzan v. Director, Missouri Department of Health, 497 U.S. 261. (1990).

Ditto, P. H., Danks, J. H., Smuker, W. D., Bookwala, J., Coppola, K. M., Dresser, R., . . . Zyzankski, S. (2001). Advance directives as acts of communication: A randomized trial. *Archives of Internal Medicine*, *161*, 421–430.

Elliott, C., & Elliott, B. (1991). From the patient's point of view: Medical ethics and the moral imagination. *Journal of Medical Ethics*, *17*, 173–178.

Fagerlin, A., & Schneider, C. E. (2004). Enough: The failure of the living will. *Hastings Center Report*, *34*(2), 30–43.

Gerhart, K. A., & Corbet, B. (1995). Uninformed consent: Biased decision making following spinal cord injury. *HEC Forum*, *7*(2–3), 110–121.

Gerhart, K. A., Joziol-McLain, J., Lowenstein, S. R., & Whiteneck, G. G. (1994). Quality of life following spinal cord injury: Knowledge and attitudes of emergency care providers. *Annals of Emergency Medicine*, *23*(4), 807–812.

Gonella, S., Campagna, S., Basso, I., Grazia De Marinis, M., & Di Giulio, P. (2019). Mechanisms by which end-of-life communication influences palliative-oriented care in nursing homes: A scoping review. *Patient Education and Counseling, 109*(12), 2134–2144. https://doi.org/10.1016/j.pec.2019.06.018

Grant, M. S., Back, A., & Dettmar, N. S. (2020). Public perceptions of advance care planning, palliative care, and hospice: A scoping review. *Journal of Palliative Medicine, 24*(1), 46–52. https://doi.org/10.1089/jpm.2020.0111

Grisso, T., & Appelbaum, P. S. (1998). *Assessing competence to consent to treatment: A guide for physicians and other health professionals*. Oxford University Press.

Health care surrogate act, Ill. Stat. § 755 ILCSD 40/. (1998). Illinois Compiled Statutes. https://www.ilga.gov/legislation/ilcs/ilcs3.asp?ActID=2111&ChapterID=60

Institute of Medicine. (2012). *Crisis standards of care: A systems framework for catastrophic disaster response: Volume 1—Introduction and CSC framework*. National Academies Press. https://doi.org/10.17226/13351

Janssen, A. L., & MacLeod, R. D. (2010). What can people approaching death teach us about how to care? *Patient Education and Counseling, 81*, 251–256. http://dx.doi.org/10.1016/j.pec.2010.02.009

Jayes, M., & Palmer, R. (2014). Initial evaluation of the consent support tool: A structured procedure to facilitate the inclusion and engagement of people with aphasia in the informed consent process. *International Journal of Speech-Language Pathology, 16*(2), 159–168.

Jonsen, A. R., Siegler, M., & Winslade, W. J. (2022). *Clinical ethics: A practical approach to ethical decisions in clinical medicine* (9th ed.). McGraw-Hill.

Lagu, T., Haywood, C., Reimold, K., DeJong, C., Walker Sterling, R., & Iezzoni, L. I. (2022). 'I am not the doctor for you': Physicians' attitudes about caring for people with disabilities. *Health Affairs, 41*(10), 1387–1395. https://doi.org/10.1377/hlthaff.2022.00475

Lantos, J. (1993). Informed consent. The whole truth for patients? *Cancer, 72*(59), 2811–2815.

Leskuski, D. (2009). The speech-language pathologist. In D. Walsh (Ed.), *Palliative medicine* (pp. 279–282). Saunders Elsevier.

Linebarger, J. S., Johnson, V., Boss, R. D., & AAP Section on Hospice and Palliative Medicine. (2022). Guidance for pediatric end-of-life care. *Pediatrics, 149*(5), e2022057011. https://doi.org/10.1542/peds.2022-057011

Lo, B. (2020). *Resolving ethical dilemmas: A guide for clinicians* (6th ed). Wolters Kluwer.

Macauley, R. (2018). *Ethics in palliative care: A complete guide*. Oxford University Press.

Mairs, N. (1996). *Waist-high in the world: A life among the nondisabled*. Beacon.

Mannix, K. (2018). *With the end in mind*. Little, Brown, Spark.

Mannix, K. (2022). *Listen: How to find the words for tender conversations*. William Collins.

Mitchell, S. L., Tetroe, J., & O'Connor, A. M. (2001). A decision aid for long-term tube feeding in cognitively impaired older persons. *Journal of the American Geriatrics Society, 49*(3), 313–316.

National Conference of Commissioners on Uniform State Laws. (1994). *Uniform health-care decisions act*. https://www.uniformlaws.org/viewdocument/final-act-78?CommunityKey=63ac0471-5975-49b0-8a36-6a4d790a4edf

National Health Service England. (2019). *Shared decision making: Summary guide*. https://www.england.nhs.uk/wp-content/uploads/2019/01/shared-decision-making-summary-guide-v1.pdf

National Institute on Aging. (2022). *Advance care planning: Advance directives for health care*. https://www.nia.nih.gov/health/advance-care-planning-advance-directives-health-care#directives

National Institute for Health and Care Excellence (NICE). (2018). *Decision aid: Enteral (tube) feeding for people living with severe dementia*. https://www.nice.org.uk/guidance/ng97/resources/patient-decision-aid-pdf-4852697007

National POLST. (2022). *Honoring the wishes of those with serious illness and frailty*. https://polst.org/

Neher, J. O. (2004). Like a river. *Hastings Center Report, 34*(2), 9–10.

Office for Human Research Protections. (1979). *The Belmont report: Ethical principles and guidelines for the protection of human subjects research*. https://www.hhs.gov/ohrp/regulations-and-policy/belmont-report/index.html

Ottawa Hospital Research Institute (OHRI). (2022). *Patient decision aids*. https://decisionaid.ohri.ca/decaids.html

Pedersen, E. R., Neighbors, C., Tidwell, J., & Lostutter, T. W. (2011). Do undergraduate student research participants read psychological research consent forms? Examining memory effects, condition effects, and individual differences. *Ethics & Behavior, 21*(4), 332–350.

Pianosi, K., Gorodzinsky, A. Y., MacLaren Chorney, J., Corsten, G., Johnson, L. B., & Hong, P. (2016). Informed consent in pediatric otolaryngology: What risks and benefits do parents recall? *Otolaryngology–Head and Neck Surgery, 155*(2), 332–229.

Pollens, R., Hillenbrand, K. L., & Sharp, H. M. (2009). Dysphagia. In D. Walsh (Ed.), *Palliative medicine* (pp. 871–876). Saunders Elsevier.

President's Commission for the Study of Ethical Problems in Medicine and Biomedical and Behavioral Research. (1983). *Deciding to forego life-sustaining treatment: A report on the ethical, medical, and legal issues in treatment decisions.* U.S. Government Publishing Office.

Rapoport, A., Shaheed, J., Newman, C., Rugg, M., & Steele, R. (2013). Parental perceptions of forgoing artificial nutrition and hydration during end-of-life care. *Pediatrics, 131*(5), 861–869.

Roehr, B. (2021). Assisted dying around the world. *BMJ, 374*, n2200. http://dx.doi.org/10.1136/bmj.n2200

Ross, L. F. (1998). *Children, families, and health care decision making*. Oxford University Press.

Sachs, G. A. (2000). Assessing decision-making capacity. *Topics in Stroke Rehabilitation, 7*(1), 62–64. https://doi.org/10.1310/UK35-Y055-1UDB-6AX5

Sahgal, S., Yande, A., Thompson, B. B., Chen, E. P., Fagerlin, A., Morgenstern, L. B., & Zahuranec, D. B. (2021). Surrogate satisfaction with decision making after intracerebral hemorrhage. *Neurocritical Care, 34*, 193–200.

Salgo v. Leland Stanford, Jr. University Board of Trustees. (Calif. Ct. App. 1957). https://caselaw.findlaw.com/court/ca-court-of-appeal/1759823.html

Schloendorff v. Society of New York Hospital. (N.Y. Ct. App. 1914). https://case-law.vlex.com/vid/schloendorff-v-soc-of-885748724

Sharp, H. M. (2015). Informed consent in clinical and research settings: What do patients and families need to make informed decisions? *Perspectives, 24*, 130–139.

Shalowitz, D. I., Garrett-Mayer, E., & Wendler, D. (2006). The accuracy of surrogate decision makers: A systematic review. *Archives Internal Medicine, 166*(5), 493–497. https://doi.org/10.1001/archinte.166.5.493

Sherlock, A., & Brownie, S. (2014). Patients' recollection and understanding of informed consent: A literature review. *ANZ Journal of Surgery, 84*, 207–210.

Shuster, E. (1997). Fifty years later: The significance of the Nuremberg Code. *New England Journal of Medicine, 337*(20), 1436–1440. https://www.nejm.org/doi/full/10.1056/nejm199711133372006

Sigman, G. S., & O'Connor, C. (1991). Exploration for physicians of the mature minor doctrine. *Journal of Pediatrics, 119*(4), 520–525.

Smuker, W. D., Houts, R. M., Danks, J. H., Ditto, P. H., Fagerlin, A., & Coppola, K. M. (2000). Modal preferences predict elderly patients' life-sustaining treatment choices as well as patients' chosen surrogates do. *Medical Decision Making, 20*, 271–280.

Spalding, R. (2021). Accuracy in surrogate end-of-life medical decision making: A critical review. *Applied Psychology: Health and Well-Being, 13*(1), 3–33. https://doi.org/10.1111/aphw.12221

Sprik, P., & Gentile, D. (2020). Cultural humility: A way to reduce LGBTQ health disparities at the end of life. *American Journal of Hospice and Palliative Medicine, 37*(6), 404–408.

Stein, J., & Brady Wagner, L. C. (2006). Is informed consent a "yes or no" response? Enhancing the shared decision-making process for persons with aphasia. *Topics in Stroke Rehabilitation, 13*, 42–46.

United States Department of Education. (2017). *Individuals with disabilities education act, Section 300.321: IEP team.* https://sites.ed.gov/idea/regs/b/d/300.321

Vincent, J.-L. (2005). Withdrawing may be preferable to withholding. *BMC Critical Care, 9*(3),

226–229. https://www.ncbi.nlm.nih.gov/pmc/articles/PMC1175874/

Wendler, D., & Rid, A. (2011). Systematic review: The effect on surrogates of making treatment decisions for others. *Annals Internal Medicine, 154*(5), 336–346.

World Medical Association. (1964). *Declaration of Helsinki.* https://www.wma.net/wp-content/uploads/2018/07/DoH-Jun1964.pdf

Yadav, K. N., Gabler, N. B., Cooney, K., Kent, S., Kim J., Herbst, N., . . . Courtright, K. R. (2017). Approximately one in three US adults completes any time of advance directive for end-of-life care. *Health Affairs, 36*(7), 1244–1251.

Zahuranec, D. B., Anspach, R. R., Roney, M. E., Fuhrel-Forbis, A., Connochie, D. M., Chen, E. P., . . . Fagerlin, A. (2018). Surrogate decision makers' perspectives on family members' prognosis after intracerebral hemorrhage. *Journal of Palliative Care, 21*(7), 965–962.

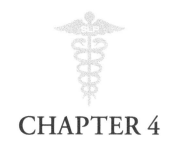

CHAPTER 4

Communication and Cognition Management for Adults With Life-Limiting Conditions

Amanda Stead and Michelle Bourgeois

> *"Endings matter, not just for the person but, perhaps even more, for the ones left behind."* —Atul Gawande, 2014

INTRODUCTION

Intuitively, communication is essential as people near the end of life (EoL). However, speech-language pathology services to support communication and cognition are often overlooked. When speech-language pathologists (SLPs) are consulted, referrals are more often related to dysphagia. In this chapter, we will discuss how SLPs can support effective communication for patients, families, and members of the professional health care team. Speech-language consultations, evaluations, and interventions for patients nearing the EoL may differ from traditional rehabilitation-focused services in focus, scope, and number of encounters. However, the SLP's knowledge and skills in assessment and treatment planning associated with speech, language, and cognition apply as they do across populations and settings (Pollens, 2004).

When people are nearing the EoL, they desire connection and the opportunity to say goodbye, resolve unfinished business, and consider their legacy (Kuhl et al., 2010; Pollens, 2004). In this chapter, we will also explore why communication is essential for people near the EoL and identify diagnostic groups of patients who often benefit from speech-language pathology services, common barriers to communication near the EoL, considerations for assessment, and examples of intervention strategies.

ESSENTIAL ROLE FOR COMMUNICATION IN END-OF-LIFE CARE

Health-Related Quality of Life (HRQL) is defined as "an individual's or a group's perceived physical and mental health over time"

(Centers for Disease Control and Prevention [CDC], 2021). HRQL relates to general well-being and a person's perception that their life is going well. Ghoshal and colleagues (2016) affirmed that physical, emotional, and social well-being are all impacted by one's medical condition or treatment and perceived HRQL and well-being. Many patients nearing the EoL have impaired communicative and/or cognitive abilities related to generalized decline and weakness, underlying disease, existing communication disorders, or a combination of these.

Poor communication diminishes patient participation in medical decisions and the patient's ability to demonstrate their capacity to make decisions. Communication is essential to both the quality and quantity of social interactions. Through the support of communication near the EoL, SLPs can impact both quality of communication and decision making, thus increasing the likelihood of the patient achieving a "good death." SLPs can support patients and families nearing EoL by ensuring accessible communication for the dual purposes of maintaining a connection with family and friends and participating in medical decisions, including symptom management (Pollens, 2020). Wallace (2013) indicated myriad reasons communication intervention is warranted for patients nearing the EoL, including (a) understanding the scope and terms of the medical situation, (b) conversations with family and the care team about the impact of the situation, and (c) communicating emotional, spiritual, and physical care needs as health status changes occur, sometimes daily. Patients who have impaired communication near the EoL are at risk of losing autonomy in a critical period of rapid change in clinical status and when multiple decisions may need to be made. Even when patients have previously stated preferences for EoL care or have completed an advance directive, these preferences often reflect hypothetical situations. Advance care planning does not account for the lived experience and specific scenarios associated with the EoL. As a result, ongoing communication about preferences is essential for patients near the EoL.

There has been increasing interest in the role of SLPs in supporting patients' communication and ability to make medical decisions (Lambert, 2012; Stead & McDonnell, 2015). SLPs and other allied health professionals who have relationships with patients may have insight into their patients' desired treatments, values, and expectations due to the strong relationships formed across therapy sessions. These relationships may place allied health professionals, including SLPs, in an ideal position to support a patient's decision making about communication, nutrition, hydration, and other needs (Chahda et al., 2017; Lambert, 2012). In addition, SLPs may help the patient and family articulate their preferences through advance care plans, which may include decisions about resuscitation, preference for location of care, and completion of advance directive documents (see also Chapters 1 and 3).

There is little literature focused on the outcomes of SLP interventions in EoL care (Chang & Bourgeois, 2020; Pollens, 2004, 2012, 2020; Wallace, 2013); however, literature in this area is emerging, and the variability in the patterns and extent of functional decline at the EoL complicates its development (Lunney et al., 2003; Toner & Shadden, 2012). SLPs can facilitate medical participation by ensuring patients can communicate with the medical care team and their loved ones. Limited or atypical communication presents a risk that the professional care team will assume the patient lacks the capacity for decision making. SLPs can ensure professionals and families receive education about how to provide information to the patient to maximize their comprehension and to support the patient's responses and ability to express their preferences.

Populations at Risk

As patients near the EoL, the combined impact of the disease progression, medication side effects, fatigue, shortness of breath, and generalized weakness all contribute to reduced communication efficacy across diagnoses. Several populations are at particularly high risk for communication or cognitive disorders near the EoL. Although the conditions we identify below are among the most common cognitive and/or communication disorders associated with palliative, hospice, or general EoL care needs, the considerations related to communication, assessment, and intervention that follow can be applied across patients and families who experience communication barriers near the EoL.

Progressive Neurologic Motor Degenerative Disorders

Progressive neurologic motor disorders, including amyotrophic lateral sclerosis (ALS), multiple sclerosis (MS), and muscular dystrophies, present specific risks for poor or reduced communication as patients near the EoL. ALS is a degenerative motor neuron disease characterized by accelerating disability and respiratory dysfunction (Genuis et al., 2021). Patients with ALS often experience significant communication difficulties with or without cognitive impairments, especially as they near the EoL. The terminal nature of the disease, communication about the disease and symptom management, and advance care planning are central to the care of these patients. Given the near-universal communi-

cation impacts of ALS, SLP services are necessary to ensure the participation of the person with ALS as they near the EoL (Pino et al., 2016). Many patients with ALS may have existing supportive communication tools in place, but communication support systems will likely need to be developed if none exist. Several studies have evaluated communication support in this population for quality of life and participation, which ultimately serves EoL communication (Brownlee & Bruening, 2012; Fried-Oken & Bardach, 2005; Fried-Oken et al., 2015; Linse et al., 2018).

Multiple sclerosis (MS) is another condition that has detrimental effects on communication, impacting the quality of EoL care. MS is the most common demyelinating disease of the central nervous system. Although the presentation of this disease is highly variable, most patients present with increasing immobility, physical dysfunction, and fatigue (Strupp et al., 2014). MS is often complicated by communication, swallowing, and cognitive impairments. Research indicates that people with MS wish to have more extensive conversations about EoL care planning and an anticipated decline in function (Buecken et al., 2012). However, studies show that patients with MS are often unsatisfied with these conversations and may lack access to palliative care services that people with other life-limiting conditions receive (Golla et al., 2014). The importance of ensuring patients with MS receive education and counseling about EoL options is highlighted by the frequency with which patients with MS report they have considered physician-assisted suicide for pain management (65%) and quality-of-life considerations (50%) (Berkman et al., 1999; Marrie et al., 2017). Numerous studies have specifically evaluated communication abilities and support for patients with MS (Baylor et al., 2010; El-Wahsh et al., 2022; Feenaughty et al., 2018).

Progressive Cognitive Disorders

Patients with progressive cognitive disorders, such as dementia, may also need support to achieve their communication goals as they near the EoL. Due to the cognitive and communication deficits associated with many progressive neurocognitive disorders, communication and decision making are often impaired. Moreover, support for persons near the EoL with dementia is often made more difficult by a lack of advance care planning (Allen et al., 2003). Patients diagnosed with primary progressive aphasia have an additional barrier to EoL communication, with rapidly deteriorating language ability being the emergent symptom of the disease (Lanzi et al., 2017). Evidence has shown that although patients with progressive neurocognitive disorders demonstrate increasingly poor communication ability across their disease courses, communication support strategies can effectively support quality of life and decision making (Chang & Bourgeois, 2020; Fried-Oken et al., 2015; Pollens, 2020). Several researchers have sought to study EoL issues in this population specifically (Hickey & Bourgeois, 2018; Regan et al., 2014). One of the significant barriers to quality EoL care in persons with dementia is that it is difficult to determine whether a person with dementia is near the EoL.

Oncological Conditions

Patients with a history of cancer, particularly head and neck cancers, pose a distinctive challenge to providers in EoL care due to the impact of the disease and treatment side effects on eating, swallowing, communication, and breathing (Mayland et al., 2020). For many patients, communication is impacted by the anatomical changes in the communication system. Head and neck cancers in particular can create direct communication barriers for patients and families near the EoL. In addition, communication modalities, such as using an artificial larynx, esophageal speech, and tracheoesophageal speech, may become more challenging for patients near the EoL due to systemic weakness, fatigue, and/or cognitive changes.

Individuals With Existing Communication Impairments

Individuals with existing communication impairments, either acquired or developmental, can face particular challenges as they experience EoL care. It is well documented that many health care providers struggle to communicate with patients with communication disorders, resulting in poorer health care outcomes and reduced satisfaction with care (Bartlett et al., 2008; Baylor et al., 2019; Burns et al., 2015).

Newly acquired communication impairments, such as aphasia or traumatic brain injury, can pose significant barriers to effective communication with the care team and with family. Among individuals with long-existing communication disorders, previously effective strategies may become more difficult or ineffective as patients experience weakness, fatigue, cognitive changes, and/or medication side effects. Adults with developmental conditions, such as Down syndrome or autism, may experience deterioration of communication skills.

Those unfamiliar with communication impairments can perceive poor communication as a lack of cognitive capacity (Simmons-Mackie et al., 2010). Therefore, people may assume patients with communication disorders lack decision-making capacity or may raise questions about broader legal competence. When a patient's capacity is questioned, they are less likely to be included in decision making about their own care.

Acute Injury

SLPs in medical settings routinely assess and treat patients with sudden-onset communication disorders after trauma, acute stroke, brain injury, and/or surgery. In addition to new-onset communication disorders such as aphasia, patients may exhibit reduced consciousness related to underlying brain injury, use of medications, or restricted communication due to medical interventions such as intubation and ventilation.

The rapid decline in health associated with acute medical events means that patients and families have little time to identify and attain their goals for EoL care. Poor communication further complicates the care team's ability to explain the situation or to engage the patient in meaningful discussion about their goals and plan of care. Whether communication is limited or delayed, the presence of a communication impairment may limit the patient's access to information and ultimately reduce their opportunity to come to terms with an unexpected but impending death.

BARRIERS TO COMMUNICATION FOR INDIVIDUALS NEARING THE END OF LIFE

When considering impacts on communication for those nearing the EoL, the primary cause of the decline and the physical, medical, psychological, personal, and contextual factors that impact functional communication must be taken into account. This section will focus on complicating factors that may impact communication near the EoL.

Physical and Medical Impacts on Communication

As discussed in Chapter 1, three distinct functional decline patterns emerge near EoL for people with progressive chronic illness: (a) terminal disease trajectory, (b) organ failure trajectory, and (c) frailty. Within the terminal disease trajectory, there is steady progression of symptoms, with rapid functional decline several months before death. Several symptoms are expected near the EoL, such as pain, shortness of breath, anxiety, depression, fatigue, lethargy, agitation, nausea and vomiting, constipation, organ failure, and medication side effects; these symptoms often increase throughout the trajectory of the dying process (see Chapter 1 for further information). Pain significantly contributes to poor communication near the EoL, as severe or long-lasting pain impacts communication and cognitive ability through reduced memory and attentional capacity (Moriarty et al., 2011).

In addition, long-lasting pain increases fatigue (Hart et al., 2003). Fatigue and decreases in attention, memory, and alertness can be compounded by the medications used for pain control near the EoL. Fatigue negatively impacts patients with end-stage cancer through reduced physical, emotional, economic, and social participation (Ghoshal et al., 2016). Additionally, medical interventions such as intubation impact a patient's communication ability. Therefore, the SLP must consider the patient's underlying medical and physical status and its likely evolving nature as they work with patients near the EoL (see Chapter 1 for further information). The cumulative impact of these physical and medical factors can put patients at high risk for poor communication and cognition as well as reduced decision-making participation.

Emotional and Psychological Impacts on Communication

Emotional distress and anxiety are expected at the EoL and can become a barrier to effective communication. Patients nearing the EoL and their families experience strong emotional responses that may be symptoms of anxiety and depression (Soto-Rubio et al., 2018; Toseland et al., 1995). Anxiety and depression have been found to have a negative impact on the quality and quantity of communication (Cohen et al., 2014). Communication impairments may also exacerbate isolation and negatively impact psychosocial well-being (Palmer et al., 2019). The effect of the emotional state on communication cannot be understated.

Social, Cultural, and Religious Impacts on Communication

One major influencing factor on a patient's experience at the EoL is the context in which they find themselves while dying. A wide range of sociocultural conditions impact health and patient-perceived outcomes. Social determinants of health correspond with how individuals are likely to be served by medical systems as they die.

Social determinants of health include geographic region, race, ethnicity, health literacy, socioeconomic status, and others (Koroukian et al., 2017). Personal health literacy is defined as "the degree to which individuals have the ability to find, understand, and use information and services to inform health-related decisions and actions for themselves and others" (CDC, 2022). Reduced or poor personal health literacy poses a barrier to communication and outcomes. For example, in one study, patients with poor personal health literacy were more likely to choose aggressive interventions rather than comfort care when provided with only verbal descriptions of the expected clinical trajectory of a patient with advanced dementia (Volandes, 2008).

Medical professionals and clinicians working with those near the EoL can achieve better communication for all patients and families by reducing use of medical jargon,

using multiple modalities to communicate, limiting reliance on written communication, and using teach-back methods to ensure comprehension (Ladin et al., 2018).

A person's health beliefs are often connected to their cultural background and spiritual or religious beliefs (Long, 2011). A patient's and family's perception of their illness or injury is influenced by their individually held belief systems, which are interwoven with culture, religion, spirituality, values, traditions, lived experience, and family dynamics. Spiritual well-being has been found to impact overall quality of life and physical, emotional, and functional well-being (Rego et al., 2020). Therefore, spirituality and religiosity are integral to palliative care, hospice care, and acute and chronic health care systems. Patients' capacity to communicate their personal priorities as they relate to beliefs, traditions, and values is essential as people face their death. Support for communication and cognition can provide the tools for patients to express existential fears, ask questions, and receive and understand individualized spiritual care.

SPEECH-LANGUAGE AND COGNITIVE EVALUATION FOR PATIENTS WITH TERMINAL ILLNESS

Prospective goals for patients nearing the EoL are not restorative but facilitative. This means that evaluating communication for patients nearing the EoL is a dynamic, ongoing, and flexible process. Functional communication should be the primary objective for assessment regardless of the underlying condition. The type of assessment is often guided more by the patient's clinical status and estimates of proximity to death than it is by the patient's underlying impairments.

As with all assessments of adults with communication impairments, every effort should be made to assess individual domains of function. Typically, a screening-level assessment considers the patient's receptive language; expressive language; cognition; voice quality and loudness; speech intelligibility, including motor functions for speech; and accessibility of alternative means of communication, including motor skills, vision, and reading ability. However, the evaluation must also assess immediate needs for functional communication, patient and family well-being, and comfort with strategies and external aids.

Context

A speech-language and cognitive evaluation may be requested for patients hospitalized in acute or intensive care, in residential care facilities, as outpatients, through home health agencies including hospice referrals, or in a hospice/palliative care facility. The location of the evaluation will often dictate some of the specific aspects of the evaluation, including a time frame, expectations, and access to ancillary or tertiary services. If a patient with acute trauma enters the hospital and is determined to be near the EoL, the goal of a speech-language or cognitive evaluation is to address immediate needs for the care team and family to know what the patient understands and to provide immediate communication support to allow the patient to state their preferences as they are able and/or to say goodbye. In this context, there are no expectations for ongoing intervention or long-term goals. On the other hand, if a patient enters hospice care due to terminal cancer and has several months left to live, the SLP's assessment of communication function will be more extensive to encompass both immediate and anticipated needs associated with the patient's decline in health.

Unfortunately, referrals for hospice and palliative care services are often initiated very late in the illness trajectory (Hawley, 2017). Although the medical team responds promptly to conduct their initial assessments of the core physical, psychosocial, and spiritual needs of the patient and family, secondary referrals to allied health professionals, including SLPs, may occur with limited time available to assess and implement a plan of care to support communication and/or cognition. Therefore, the SLP who responds to such consults will often need to implement recommendations very quickly. It is common that the point of entry for speech-language referrals is dysphagia, even when the patient has evident communication impairments. Every SLP should incorporate communication and cognitive needs in the assessment of every patient.

Caregivers

Caregivers serve an essential function for patients near the EoL. Their roles are so deeply interwoven with the experience of death that both palliative care and hospice service dedicate specific resources to support families and caregivers during this time. It is essential to assess both caregiver experience and well-being, as caregivers will often bear the responsibility of communication support for the patient. Several tools can be embedded directly or indirectly alongside assessment to help the clinician determine the caregiver's capacity for intervention support. See Table 4–1 for suggested caregiver assessment tools.

Alongside more formal questionnaires or survey assessments of caregivers, informal interviews of caregivers serve an essential role in informing the SLP about the patient's needs and concurrently assessing the caregiver's skills in observation and as a communication partner. Caregivers will likely appreciate the opportunity to report communication barriers

Table 4–1. Selected Caregiver Burden Assessment Tools

Tool	Population	Description
Caregiver's Burden Scale in End-of-Life Care (Dumont et al., 2008)	Family/caregivers of patients with terminal cancer	16-item tool that explicitly assesses family/caregivers' burden within the palliative care context
Caregiver Reaction Assessment (Petrinec et al., 2016)	Caregivers of patients receiving palliative care	24-item tool to assess overall caregiver burden across multiple domains, including feelings of role captivity, overload, competence, personal gain, coping, family beliefs and conflict, job conflicts, and financial disruption
Family Appraisal of Caregiving Questionnaire for Palliative Care (Cooper et al., 2005)	Caregivers of patients receiving palliative care	26-item measure of a family's self-appraisal of caregiving that can be used in clinical assessment
Zarit Burden Inventory (Zarit et al., 1980)	Caregivers	22-item self-report of caregiver burden, role strain, and personal strain
Grief Experience Questionnaire (Barrett & Scott, 1989)	Bereaved spouses	Self-administered questionnaire measuring various components of grief following the death of a loved one
Marwit–Meuser Caregiver Grief Inventory (Marwit et al., 2007)	Caregivers of people with dementia, acquired brain injury, and cancer	18- to 50-item inventory designed to measure the grief experience of family caregivers
Bereavement Risk Index (BRI; Kristjanson et al., 2005)	Family members anticipating loss	4-item measurement administered by allied health professionals to determine if family members should be classified as high, medium, or low risk for difficult grief reactions

and inform the SLP about strategies they have already tried, their ideas, and what they may find overwhelming. Some examples of helpful questions to include in the patient/caregiver interview are:

- "Why don't we start by telling me what you already know (or think is happening) and understand, and we will go from there?"
- "What are your goals for your loved ones' communication during this time?"
- "Are there particular challenges you see in their ability to communicate?"

- "What is something I could do to support you and your loved one to have quality interactions at this time?"
- "Is there anything that [name of the patient] seems to want to communicate but cannot?"

Direct Assessment

Direct assessment can collect information about the patient's overall clinical status and identify primary areas of communication impairments and needs. Due to the vast array of potential areas of impact for a patient near the EoL, the SLP must choose assessment tools that best reflect the patient's most urgent communication needs. In addition, the SLP will often have limited time with the patient because other professionals will also be engaged in the person's care, family caregivers and visitors may take priority, and the patient may have limited periods of alertness. Therefore, the speech-language and cognitive assessment must be conducted efficiently. Before the assessment, the clinician can set the assessment up for success by considering several patient and environmental factors that may impact the assessment outcome.

enter the assessment with a clear idea of the main areas of focus for assessment. Where possible, a brief discussion or interview with primary professionals (e.g., primary nurse or social worker) who have seen the patient recently, as well as primary family caregivers, will inform the SLP. Through this interview, the SLP will gain information about the patient's general level of alertness, the time of day the patient is likely to be awake and alert, physical status and capacity for sitting upright and for how long, and primary communication needs. This preparation ensures the SLP has the appropriate assessment tools and trial therapy strategies available and can conduct the assessment efficiently. Both primary and secondary areas should be evaluated before setting goals and choosing intervention approaches. Below is a suggested outline of assessment for patients nearing the EoL.

Tips to Set Up Your Assessment for Success

- Consider the patient's medication schedule and the impact their medications may have on their alertness or pain status.
- Eliminate background noise including music, television, and nonessential alarms.
- It is ideal to have one or two key family caregivers present or contributing to the interview and assessment, but encourage other visitors to sit out during the assessment.
- Modify the patient's position to best serve the desired outcomes of the evaluation.
- If the evaluation is for eating or swallowing, schedule near mealtime and offer foods that the patient prefers.

Based on the patient's primary diagnosis and medical history review, the SLP should

---

Steps for Assessment of Communication in Patients Nearing the End of Life

1. Medical Record Review: Establish primary diagnosis, secondary diagnoses, current medical status, medications, and a time frame and nature of decline anticipated when possible. Contact relevant team members, including nurse and/or social worker or source of referral, to clarify goals of the referral and known concerns for the patient and/or family caregivers.

2. Interview: Determine patient and family goals for care and current difficulties.

3. Assess Communication Function:
   a. Functional communication overall

b. Assess domains of speech-language and cognition:

   i. Speech intelligibility

   ii. Receptive and expressive language

   iii. Cognition

   iv. Voice quality and loudness

   v. Oral mechanism/cranial nerve function

4. Assess Secondary Areas:

   a. Well-being

   b. Grief

   c. Depression

   d. Caregiver burden/coping

   e. Vision and hearing

   f. Gross motor skills (ambulatory, able to sit up)

   g. Fine motor skills (able to manipulate technology or low-tech AAC, able to point)

5. Discuss Goals:

   a. Patient's expressed goals

   b. Family caregivers' expressed goals and needs for communication

   c. Professional care team members' expressed goals and needs for communication

6. Trial Therapy:

   a. External supports (signage, hearing assistive technology, environmental modifications, etc.)

   b. Low- or high-tech AAC

   c. Compensatory strategies

   d. Caregiver training

Several assessment tools have been developed to capture functional communication holistically. See Table 4–2 for examples of functional communication assessments. Functional communication may also be assessed through conversations, language samples, or patient observation during caregiver or medical professional interactions. Through these informal methods, clinicians can glean information about the patient's ability to: (a) follow directions, (b) request information or support, (c) choose between options, and (d) recall information from events that have already happened.

Indirect Assessment

Several indirect assessment methods can be used to evaluate the function and status of a patient near the EoL. Although indirect assessment methods, such as caregiver questionnaires, can be impacted by the informant's personality, mood, and burden level, research indicates that functional impairments may be captured better via indirect methods than through direct assessment in a given session (Lima-Silva et al., 2015). Both patient and caregiver interview questions can support indirect assessment by targeting urgent concerns or immediate struggles. In addition, indirect assessments are a tool to collect information about patient preferences, practices, well-being, and spirituality. See Table 4–3 for examples.

INTERVENTION PLANS

Functional Goals and Outcomes

When writing goals for patients near the EoL, the goals must be appropriate for the patient's declining status. Taking an outcomes-focused

Table 4–2. Selected Functional Communication Assessment Tools

Tool	Population	Description
Revised Edinburgh Functional Communication Profile (REFCP; Wirz et al., 1990)	Adults with speech, language, and cognitive/communication impairments	Assesses functional communication via both verbal and nonverbal modalities
ASHA Functional Assessment of Communication Skills (ASHA FACS; Fratalli et al., 1995)	Adults with speech, language, and cognitive/communication impairments	Assesses functional communication via both verbal and nonverbal modalities
Functional Communication Profile–Revised (FCP-R; Kleiman, 2003)	Children 3 years old through adults with communication impairments	Assesses an overall inventory of the individual's communication abilities, mode of communication, and degree of independence
FLACC (Face, Legs, Activity, Cry, Consolability) Pain Scale (Voepel-Lewis et al., 1997)	Children starting at 2 months of age through 7 years old and can be used for individuals who are unable to communicate their pain	Assesses pain through nonverbal communication
Communication Effectiveness Index (CETI; Lomas et al., 1989)	Adults with acquired communication impairments	Assesses nonverbal communication ability
Voice Handicap Index (Jacobson et al., 1997)	Adults with acquired voice impairments	Assesses the biopsychosocial impact of a voice disorder

Table 4–3. Selected Grief and Spirituality Assessment Tools

Tool	Population
Beck Hopelessness Scale (Beck, 1988)	Ethnically diverse U.S. population; validated in palliative care population
Brief Grief Questionnaire (Shear et al., 2006)	Bereaved community-dwelling adults
Spirit Screening (Maugans, 1996)	Persons with chronic illness or in palliative care
Spiritual Relationship Model (Lartey, 1997)	Multifaith and crosscultural for palliative care
Spiritual Assessment Questions (Anandarajah & Hight, 2001)	Persons with stroke, cancer, disability, and chronic illness
Brief Spiritual Beliefs Inventory (SBI-15; Holland et al., 1998)	Multifaith measure of individuals with religious and spiritual beliefs and practices

Case 1

José is a 74-year-old bilingual cisgender male with malignant neoplasm of the frontal lobe. A medical record review includes history of severe expressive aphasia, moderate receptive aphasia, mild dysphagia, severe apraxia, hemiplegia, and hemiparesis. The SLP assesses José using a quick aphasia battery and informal assessment because he becomes highly agitated when asked questions. The patient's immediate needs include participation in medical decision making. Caregiver training in communication strategies to support the patient's communication is a primary focus.

Sample goals:

- Patient will demonstrate increased attempts to communicate wants, needs, and decisions using visual support and caregiver assistance.
- The caregiver will demonstrate supportive communication strategies [specify one or two] with patient within 90% of communication attempts to increase patient ability to communicate wants and needs.
- Patient will demonstrate the ability to point to body parts accurately in 80% of trials to communicate the site of pain or discomfort.

approach, SLPs should prioritize the patient's and family's goals and participation. A primary focus is to allow the patient to indicate medical status, participate in decision making, manage affairs, and engage with caregivers and family. Goals should support family connection, socialization, spirituality, grief processing, and life review. As the intervention is planned, the patient burden should be minimized by focusing on facilitative and/or compensatory strategies rather than rehabilitative-focused strategies.

Goals should reflect the needs and type of intervention used. Below is a list of goal examples and formats that can be adapted to serve patients near the EoL.

For sample goals below, relevant or patient-specific goals should be tailored.

- Patient will use visual supports to express symptoms and concerns for end-of-life care in [#] of [#] opportunities.
- Patient will use visual supports to participate in medical decision making in [#] of [#] opportunities.
- Patient will demonstrate gestures or nonverbal communication within [#] of [#] opportunities to promote energy conservation with mild verbal/visual cues or prompts.

- A personalized communication board will be collaboratively developed with patient and family, with [#] key topics and [#] keywords on each page.
- The patient will complete [#] successful exchanges with the communication partner in [#] minutes or less [baseline # exchange in # min].
- The client will be able to share [#] personal stories about themselves, using personalized communication aid through [type training], on [#/#] practices in therapy.

- The patient will increase communication participation activities using alternative communication options identified in therapy, including safety alerts, starting a new topic, and choosing TV channels.
- [Patient/Caregiver] will demonstrate improved communication success as measured by an improved score on the Communication Effectiveness Survey [baseline score #/#] after participating in education with SLP.

- The patient and SLP will collaboratively develop personalized cognitive and communication support for improved function with [activity], to compensate for [deficit area]. Success will be measured by [outcomes measure].
- Using Self-Anchored Rating Scale, [caregiver/family] will improve rating of communication skill from baseline of [X/10] after [#] weeks with SLP collaboration to implement specific supportive communication strategies.

Alternative or Augmented Communication (AAC)

Even when a patient's communication system is not affected directly by disease or disorder, the associated physical symptoms of EoL, such as pain and lethargy, can detrimentally impact communication and warrant intervention. However, hospice and palliative care referrals for dysphagia management far outweigh other SLP referrals for communication interventions (Hawley, 2017). AAC use in EoL care can support patients in living as fully as possible until death. Furthermore, integrating psychological and spiritual aspects of care can offer an additional support system to help the families cope during the patient's decline and bereavement (Pollens, 2020). Finally, AAC can help patients meet goals near the EoL, including communications for quality of life and medical decision making.

Pollens (2020) explained that one use of the most basic forms of AAC, written communication, may provide individuals access to pain relief and other forms of comfort. AAC can also serve as a form of energy conservation (Fried-Oken & Bardach, 2005), so offering alternative support for communication can allow patients and families to continue to

connect. Providing easily accessible paper and pencils, whiteboards, alphabet charts, a simple board with basic care vocabulary, or picture boards can make it easy for patients to express their essential needs. Hurtig and Downey (2008) have shown a positive relationship between client responsiveness and care when using AAC.

When offering AAC support to patients and families, several factors should be considered, including (a) patient preference, (b) baseline and immediacy of implementation, (c) expected time frame of use, and (d) training and implementation issues. Finally, any AAC intervention must consider the presumptive decline of sensory systems, mobility, cognition, and patient and caregiver energy required for continued use. High-tech AAC devices may not be the most appropriate for the EoL population because of the burdens associated with new learning and the complexities of physical accessibility. Individuals who are already AAC users and their families report that the complexity of high-tech AAC devices can become a barrier during the EoL period (Fried-Oken & Bardach, 2005). In addition, due to the complex nature of programming and training for many high-tech AAC devices, medical staff and families may forgo use entirely, depriving the patient of an accessible communication system (Hurtig & Downey, 2008). When patients are nearing the EoL with new and critical symptoms that impact communication, low-tech alternative means of communication, such as simple communication boards, may be more easily implemented. See Figure 4–1 for an example of a low-tech AAC board for communication in EoL care.

In addition to supporting social connection, AAC can support individuals' participation in medical and EoL decision making. For example, research has shown that with visual aids, persons with dementia demonstrated significantly better understanding, reasoning, and appreciation of complex choices, each of which extends the patient's capacity to participate in decisions about their care (Chang & Bourgeois, 2020). See Figure 4–2 for examples of simple choice boards to support decision making (see Appendix B for further examples).

When patients and families face a significant change in function or rapid decline, the universal nature of low-tech communication boards and their ease of implementation can immediately increase the quality of communication and participation. Whichever form of AAC intervention is implemented with a patient, the tools must have both adaptability and longevity across the continuum of the patient's decline.

Role of Supported Communication and Caregiver Training

Caregivers are an integral part of EoL care. Caregiver preparedness helps reduce some

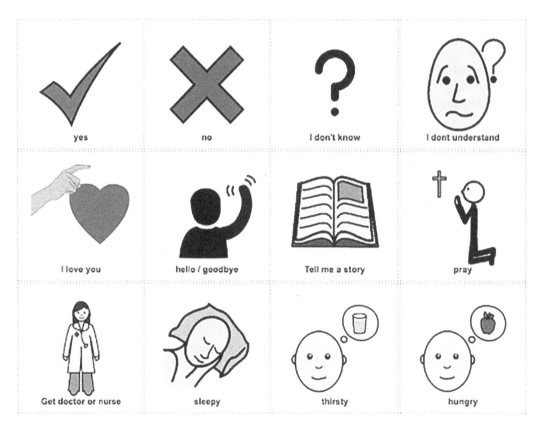

Figure 4–1. Example low-tech AAC board.

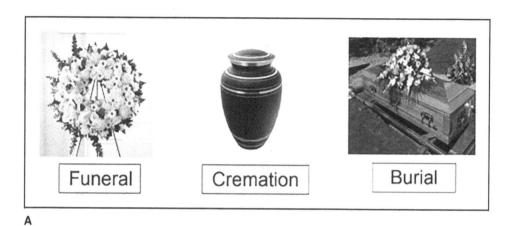

A

B

Figure 4–2. A. Example low-tech AAC board to aid with funeral planning. **B.** Example low-tech AAC board to aid with personal affairs planning.

negative impacts associated with caring for someone near the EoL, including fear, stress, and anxiety (Williams, 2018). When possible, SLPs should involve the primary caregivers in setting goals to meet both the patient's and caregivers' goals for communication. If caregivers see the benefit of the communication strategies, it will likely increase generalization and enhance the patient's communication throughout the dying process. For example, if a low-tech AAC board is implemented for essential social communication, caregivers should be taught how to present, navigate, and update the board as necessary. In addition, several teaching strategies can be used to train caregivers to interact better with their loved ones near the EoL. Basic approaches to caregiver training often include training the caregiver to use communication strategies such as visual communication aids, swallowing strategies, and environmental modifications.

Supported conversation (Kagan, 1998), a strategy initially developed to aid communication with persons with aphasia, provides many tenets that are equally applicable to people near the EoL:

- speak in a normal tone of voice;
- acknowledge communication difficulties and try to repair them;
- write keywords and keep a written log of the conversation that can be reviewed;
- use a drawing or supportive gestures; and
- ask yes/no questions to confirm understanding.

Other strategies for caregiver training include the teach-back method (Farris, 2015) and the FOCUSED program (Ripich, 1994). These strategies are iterative communication techniques to support knowledge acquisition, understanding, and health literacy. Some example goals that feature caregiver training are provided in the following box.

- Caregivers will demonstrate clarification and summarizing strategies within 90% of opportunities to confirm understanding of patient's expressed wants, needs, thoughts, feelings, and ideas.
- Caregivers will verbally identify three supportive communication strategies to increase patient's ability to meet wants and needs after completion of communication partner training session.
- Supported conversation training will be completed with the patient and caregiver/family, with each partner receiving three key strategies to practice.
- Caregivers will verbally identify three supportive communication strategies to increase patient's ability to meet wants and needs.

Several other direct and indirect interventions can be used with patients near the EoL. Intervention approaches depend on the patient's underlying impairment, communication needs, context, and trajectory of decline. Table 4–4 outlines some additional suggestions for interventions based on communication and cognition needs.

Sensory impairment can also profoundly impact communication near the EoL and should be incorporated into the intervention plan. It is well known that sensory impairments compound the impact of communication impairments. For example, patients with hearing impairment should continue to use hearing aids or amplification as often as possible. In addition, prescription or "reader" glasses should be readily available, and patients with poor vision may benefit from larger font sizes, magnifiers, and brighter lighting.

Table 4–4. Potential Intervention Based on Areas of Impact

Area of Impact	Possible Interventions
Expression	• Supported communication strategies—caregiver training • Visual and written supports including low-tech communication boards • Partner-assisted scanning
Auditory comprehension	• Supported communication strategies—caregiver training • Train topic maintenance strategies such as confirming understanding and asking for clarification or repetition • Use of visual and written supports • Verify hearing status—use amplification if necessary • Eliminate environmental distractions such as television
Fatigue	• Communicate during alert times • Reduce cognitive burden during interactions through contextual supports • Prioritize communication attempts that align with patient and caregiver goals for EoL (e.g., only medical decisions, social interactions)
Pain	• Use visual aids to support patient capacity to convey pain level • Visual and written supports to help patient indicate need for pain interventions • Visual and written supports to help patients make medical decisions and verify choices • Choose communication time when pain is well-controlled
Reduced cognition	• Ensure interactions reduce cognitive taxation by reducing confrontational or memory-laden questions unless necessary • Use visual and written aids to support direct questions or communication interactions about health status or medical decisions • Eliminate environmental distractions such as television
Quality of life	• Visual supports and opportunities to discuss life review and relevant cultural, spiritual, and/or religion-specific topics • Supports to express thanks to specific people • Supports to express regret and apology to specific people • Opportunities and support to divulge personal information (e.g., passwords, location of valuables)

Importance of Communication for Dysphagia and Feeding Support

Comprehensive dysphagia management for adults nearing the EoL is addressed in Chapter 5. It is essential for SLPs who are consulted for dysphagia to incorporate communication and cognition as an essential aspect of the management of feeding and dysphagia needs as patients near the EoL. Communication support can validate the patient's understanding of safety and comfort and uphold the patient's capacity to express food and drink preferences. Given that the trajectory of dying very often includes dysphagia, patients, families, and professional care teams may encounter decisions about enhancing nutrition or swallowing support, including managing dysphagia symptoms that cause discomfort. Suppose the option of artificially administered nutrition and hydration support through tube feeding and/or intravenous hydration is presented. In that case, a direct assessment of patients' preferences to accept or forgo these interventions should be ascertained as often as possible (see Chapter 3 for further information). Case 2 illustrates the direct relationship between communication, feeding, and dysphagia management (see Chapter 5 for further information).

Case 2

Farah is a 93-year-old cisgender female with metastatic cervical cancer and moderate oral dysphagia with minimal intake. Communication and cognitive support goals focus on patient selection of preferred foods, including flavors and textures.

- Patient will select preferred food/drink items when the caregiver presents a choice among three captioned picture options.

- Patient will identify preferred food items/snacks when provided with a choice of three captioned pictures to instruct family members about foods to have available to increase pleasure associated with eating.

- Patient will verbally recall and identify five risks of diet modification requirements to demonstrate an understanding of choices.

CONCLUSION

Communication is essential for patients nearing the EoL. From a clinical care perspective, one primary goal of intervention is to maximize patients' ability to report symptoms and to participate in decision making about their care (Pollens, 2020). Functional, practical, adaptable, and accessible communication at the EoL is paramount for quality EoL care for the patient and assists the professional care team and the patient's family and friends. As patients and their families experience the process of dying, the SLP's expertise supports essential communication and patient autonomy with a lasting impact on friends and family after the patient dies.

REFERENCES

Allen, R. S., Kwak, J., Lokken, K. L., & Haley, W. E. (2003). End-of-life issues in the context of Alzheimer's disease. *Alzheimer's Care Quarterly, 4*(4), 312–330. https://www.ncbi.nlm.nih.gov/pmc/articles/PMC2789353/

Anandarajah, G., & Hight, E. (2001). Spirituality and medical practice: Using the HOPE questions as a practical tool for spiritual assessment. *American Family Physician, 63*, 81–89.

Barrett, T. W., & Scott, T. B. (1989). Development of the Grief Experience Questionnaire. *Suicide and Life-Threatening Behavior, 19*(2), 201–215. https://doi.org/10.1111/j.1943-278x.1989.tb01033.x

Bartlett, G., Blais, R., Tamblyn, R., Clermont, R. J., & MacGibbon, B. (2008). Impact of patient communication problems on the risk of preventable adverse events in acute care settings. *Canadian Medical Association Journal, 178*(12), 1555–1562.

Baylor, C., Burns, M., McDonough, K., Mach, H., & Yorkston, K. (2019). Teaching medical students skills for effective communication with patients who have communication disorders.

American Journal of Speech-Language Pathology, 28(1), 155–164. https://doi.org/10.1044/2018_AJSLP-18-0130

Baylor, C., Yorkston, K., Bamer, A., Britton, D., & Amtmann, D. (2010). Variables associated with communicative participation in people with multiple sclerosis: A regression analysis. *American Journal of Speech-Language Pathology, 5*(19), 143–153. https://doi.org/10.1044/1058-0360 (2009/08-0087)

Beck, A. T. (1988). *BHS, Beck Hopelessness Scale: Manual.* Psychological Corp., Harcourt Brace Jovanovich.

Berkman, C. S., Cavallo, P. F., Chesnut, W. C., & Holland, N. J. (1999). Attitudes toward physician-assisted suicide among persons with multiple sclerosis. *Journal of Palliative Medicine, 2*(1), 51–63. https://doi.org/10.1089/jpm.1999.2.51

Brownlee, A., & Bruening, L. M. (2012). Methods of communication at end of life for the person with amyotrophic lateral sclerosis. *Topics in Language Disorders, 32*(2), 168–185. https://doi.org/10.1097/tld.0b013e31825616ef

Buecken, R., Galushko, M., Golla, H., Strupp, J., Hahn, M., Ernstmann, N., . . . Voltz, R. (2012). Patients feeling severely affected by multiple sclerosis: How do patients want to communicate about end-of-life issues? *Patient Education and Counseling, 88*(2), 318–324. https://doi.org/10.1016/j.pec.2012.03.010

Burns, M., Baylor, C., Dudgeon, B. J., Starks, H., & Yorkston, K. (2015). Asking the stakeholders: Perspectives of individuals with aphasia, their family caregivers, and physicians regarding communication during medical interactions. *American Journal of Speech-Language Pathology, 24,* 341–357.

Centers for Disease Control and Prevention. (2021). *Health-Related Quality of Life (HRQOL).* https://www.cdc.gov/hrqol/index.htm

Centers for Disease Control and Prevention. (2022). *What is health literacy?* https://www.cdc.gov/healthliteracy/learn/index.html

Chahda, L., Mathisen, B., & Carey, L. (2017). The role of speech-language pathologists in adult palliative care. *International Journal of Speech-Language Pathology, 19*(1), 58–68. https://www.doi.org/10.1080/17549507.2016.1241301

Chang, W. D., & Bourgeois, M. S. (2020). Effects of visual aids for end-of-life care on decisional capacity of people with dementia. *American Journal of Speech-Language Pathology, 29*(1), 185–200. https://www.doi.org/10.1044/2019_AJSLP-19-0028

Cohen, A. S., McGovern, J. E., Dinzeo, T. J., & Covington, M. A. (2014). Speech deficits in serious mental illness: A cognitive resource issue? *Schizophrenia Research, 160*(1–3), 173–179.

Cooper, B., Kinsella, G. J., & Picton, C. (2005). Development and initial validation of a family appraisal of caregiving questionnaire for palliative care. *Psycho-Oncology, 15*(7), 613–622. https://doi.org/10.1002/pon.1001

Dumont, S., Fillion, L., Gagnon, P., & Bernier, N. (2008). A new tool to assess family caregivers' burden during end-of-life care. *Journal of Palliative Care, 24,* 151–161. https://doi.org/10.1177/082585970802400304

El-Wahsh, S., Balandin, S., Bogaardt, H., Kumfor, F., & Ballard, K. J. (2022). Managing communication changes in persons with multiple sclerosis: Findings from qualitative focus groups. *International Journal of Language & Communication Disorders, 57*(3), 680–694.

Farris, C. (2015). The teach back method. *Home Healthcare Now, 33*(6), 344–345.

Feenaughty, L., Tjaden, K., Weinstock-Guttman, B., & Benedict, R. H. (2018). Separate and combined influence of cognitive impairment and dysarthria on functional communication in multiple sclerosis. *American Journal of Speech-Language Pathology, 27*(3), 1051–1065.

Fratalli, C., Thompson, C., Holland, A., Wohl, C., & Ferketic, M. (1995). *Functional Assessment of Communication Skills for Adults (ASHA FACS).* American Speech-Language-Hearing Association.

Fried-Oken, M., & Bardach, L. (2005). End-of-life issues for people who use AAC. *Perspectives of the ASHA Special Interest Groups, 14*(3), 15–19. https://doi.org/10.1044/aac14.3.15

Fried-Oken, M., Mooney, A., & Peters, B. (2015). Supporting communication for patients with neurodegenerative disease. *NeuroRehabilita-tion, 37*(1), 69–87. https://doi.org/10.3233/NRE-151241

Gawande, A. (2014). *Being mortal: Medicine and what matters in the end.* Metropolitan Books.

Genuis, S. K., Luth, W., Campbell, S., Bubela, T., & Johnston, W. S. (2021). Communication about end of life for patients living with amyotrophic lateral sclerosis: A scoping review of the empirical evidence. *Frontiers in Neurology, 12.* https://doi.org/10.3389/fneur.2021.683197

Ghoshal, A., Salins, N., Deodhar, J., Damani, A., & Muckaden, M. A. (2016). Fatigue and quality of life outcomes of palliative care consultation: A prospective, observational study in a tertiary cancer center. *Indian Journal of Palliative Care, 22*(4), 416–426. https://doi.org/10.4103/0973-1075.191766

Golla, H., Galushko, M., Pfaff, H., & Voltz, R. (2014). Multiple sclerosis and palliative care—Perceptions of severely affected multiple sclerosis patients and their health professionals: A qualitative study. *BMC Palliative Care, 13*(1), 11. https://doi.org/10.1186/1472-684X-13-11

Hart, R. P., Wade, J. B., & Martelli, M. F. (2003). Cognitive impairment in patients with chronic pain: The significance of stress. *Current Pain and Headache Reports, 7*(2), 116–126. https://doi.org/10.1007/s11916-003-0021-5

Hawley, P. (2017). Barriers to access to palliative care. *Palliative Care, 10,* https://doi.org/10.1177/1178224216688887

Hickey, E., & Bourgeois, M. (2018). Quality of life and end of life issues. In E. Hickey & M. Bourgeois (Eds.), *Dementia: Person-centered assessment and intervention* (2nd ed., pp. 351–380). Taylor & Francis.

Holland, J. C., Kash, K. M., Passik, S., Gronert, M. K., Sison, A., Lederberg, M., . . . Fox, B. (1998). A Brief Spiritual Beliefs Inventory for use in quality of life research in life threatening illness. *Psycho-Oncology: Journal of the Psychological, Social and Behavioral Dimensions of Cancer, 7*(6), 460–469.

Hurtig, R. R., & Downey, D. (2008). *Augmentative and alternative communication in acute and critical care settings.* Plural Publishing.

Jacobson, B. H., Johnson, A., Grywalski, C., Silbergleit, A., Jacobson, G., Benninger, M. S., & Newman, C. W. (1997). The Voice Handicap Index (VHI) development and validation. *American Journal of Speech-Language Pathology, 6*(3), 66–70.

Kagaen, A. (1998). Supported conversation for adults with aphasia: Methods and resources for training conversation partners. *Aphasiology, 12*(9), 816–830.

Kleiman, L. I. (2003). *Functional Communication Profile Revised.* LinguiSystems.

Koroukian, S. M., Schiltz, N. K., Warner, D. F., Given, C. W., Schluchter, M., Owusu, C., & Berger, N. A. (2017). Social determinants, multimorbidity, and patterns of end-of-life care in older adults dying from cancer. *Journal of Geriatric Oncology, 8*(2), 117–124.

Kristjanson, L. J., Cousins, K., Smith, J., & Lewin, G. (2005). Evaluation of the Bereavement Risk Index (BRI): A community hospice care protocol. *International Journal of Palliative Nursing, 11*(12), 610–618.

Kuhl, D., Stanbrook, M. B., & Hébert, P. C. (2010). What people want at the end of life. *Canadian Medical Association Journal, 182*(16), 1707. https://doi.org/10.1503/cmaj.101201

Ladin, K., Buttafarro, K., Hahn, E., Koch-Weser, S., & Weiner, D. E. (2018). "End-of-life care? I'm not going to worry about that yet." Health literacy gaps and end-of-life planning among elderly dialysis patients. *The Gerontologist, 58*(2), 290–299.

Lambert, H. (2012). The allied health care professional's role in assisting medical decision making at the end of life. *Topics in Language Disorders, 32,* 119–136. http://doi.org/10.1097/TLD.0b013e318254d321

Lanzi, A., Burshnic, V., & Bourgeois, M. (2017). Person-centered memory and communication strategies for adults with dementia. *Topics in Language Disorders, 37*(4), 361–374. https://doi.org/10.1097/TLD.0000000000000136

Lartey, A. (1997). *In living color: An intercultural approach to personal care and counseling.* Jessica Kingsley Publishers.

Lima-Silva, T. B., Bahia, V. S., Carvalho, V. A., Guimarães, H. C., Caramelli, P., Balthazar, M. L. F., . . . Yassuda, M. S. (2015). Direct and indirect assessments of activities of daily living in behavioral variant frontotemporal dementia and Alzheimer disease. *Journal of Geriatric Psychiatry and Neurology, 28*(1), 19–26.

Linse, K., Aust, E., Joos, M., & Hermann, A. (2018). Communication matters—Pitfalls and promise of hightech communication devices in palliative care of severely physically disabled patients with amyotrophic lateral sclerosis. *Frontiers in Neurology, 9*, 603. https://doi.org/10.3389/fneur.2018.00603

Lomas, J., Pickard, L., Bester, S., Elbard, H., Finlayson, A., & Zoghaib, C. (1989). The Communicative Effectiveness Index: Development and psychometric evaluation of a functional communication measure for adult aphasia. *Journal of Speech and Hearing Disorders, 54*(1), 113–124.

Long, C. O. (2011). Cultural and spiritual considerations in palliative care. *Journal of Pediatric Hematology/Oncology, 33*, S96–S101.

Lunney, J. R., Lynn, J., Foley, D. J., Lipson, S., & Guralnik, J. M. (2003). Patterns of functional decline at the end of life. *Journal of the American Medical Association, 289*(18), 2387–2392.

Marrie, R. A., Salter, A., Tyry, T., Cutter, G., Cofield, S., & Fox, R. (2017). High hypothetical interest in physician-assisted death in multiple sclerosis. *Neurology, 88*(16), 1528–1534. https://doi.org/10.1212/WNL.0000000000003831

Marwit, S. J., Chibnall, J. T., Dougherty, R., Jenkins, C., & Shawgo, J. (2007). Assessing pre-death grief in cancer caregivers using the Marwit–Meuser Caregiver Grief Inventory (MM-CGI). *Psycho-Oncology, 17*(3), 300–303. https://doi.org/10.1002/pon.1218

Maugans, T. (1996). The SPIRITual history. *Archives of Family Medicine, 5*, 11–15.

Mayland, C. R., Ho, Q. M., Doughty, H. C., Rogers, S. N., Peddinti, P., Chada, P., . . . Dey, P. (2020). The palliative care needs and experiences of people with advanced head and neck cancer: A scoping review. *Palliative Medicine, 35*(1), 27–44. https://doi.org/10.1177/0269216320963892

Moriarty, O., McGuire, B. E., & Finn, D. P. (2011). The effect of pain on cognitive function: A review of clinical and preclinical research. *Progress in Neurobiology, 93*(3), 385–404. https://doi.org/10.1016/j.pneurobio.2011.01.002

Palmer, A. D., Carder, P. C., White, D. L., Saunders, G., Woo, H., Graville, D. J., & Newsom, J. T. (2019). The impact of communication impairments on the social relationships of older adults: Pathways to psychological well-being. *Journal of Speech, Language, and Hearing Research, 62*(1), 1–21.

Petrinec, A., Burant, C., & Douglas, S. (2016). Caregiver reaction assessment: Psychometric properties in caregivers of advanced cancer patients. *Psycho-Oncology, 26*(6), 862–865. https://doi.org/10.1002/pon.4159

Pino, M., Parry, R., Land, V., Faull, C., Feathers, L., & Seymour, J. (2016). Engaging terminally ill patients in end of life talk: How experienced palliative medicine doctors navigate the dilemma of promoting discussions about dying. *PloS ONE, 11*(5). https://doi.org/10.1371/journal.pone.0156174

Pollens, R. (2004). Role of the speech-language pathologist in palliative hospice care. *Journal of Palliative Medicine, 7*(5), 694–702.

Pollens, R. (2020). Facilitating client ability to communicate in palliative end-of-life care. *Topics in Language Disorders, 40*(3), 264–277. https://doi.org/10.1097/tld.0000000000000220

Pollens, R. D. (2012). Integrating speech-language pathology services in palliative end-of-life care. *Topics in Language Disorders, 32*(2), 137–148.

Regan, A., Tapley, M., & Jolley, D. (2014). Improving end of life care for people with dementia. *Nursing Standard, 28*(48), 37–43. https://pubmed.ncbi.nlm.nih.gov/25074121/

Rego, F., Gonçalves, F., Moutinho, S., Castro, L., & Nunes, R. (2020). The influence of spirituality on decision-making in palliative care outpatients: A cross-sectional study. *BMC Palliative Care, 19*(1), 1–14.

Ripich, D. (1994). Functional communication with AD patients: A caregiver training program. *Alzheimer's Disease and Associated Disorders, 8*(3), 95–109.

Simmons-Mackie, N., Raymer, A., Armstrong, E., Holland, A., & Cherney, L. R. (2010). Communication partner training in aphasia: A systematic review. *Archives of Physical Medicine and Rehabilitation, 91*(12), 1814–1837.

Shear, K. M., Jackson, C. T., Essock, S. M., Donahue, S. A., & Felton, C. J. (2006). Brief Grief Questionnaire. *Psychiatric Services.*

Soto-Rubio, A., Perez-Marin, M., Tomas Miguel, J., & Barreto Martin, P. (2018). Emotional distress of patients at end-of-life and their caregivers: Interrelation and predictors. *Frontiers in Psychology, 9*, 2199.

Stead, A., & McDonnell, C. (2015). Discussing end of life care: An opportunity. *Perspectives of the ASHA Special Interest Groups, 20*(1), 12–15. https://doi.org/10.1044/gero20.1.12

Strupp, J., Romotzky, V., Galushko, M., Golla, H., & Voltz, R. (2014). Palliative care for severely affected patients with multiple sclerosis: When and why? Results of a Delphi survey of health care professionals. *Journal of Palliative Medicine, 17*(10), 1128–1136. https://doi.org/10.1089/jpm.2013.0667

Toner, M. A., & Shadden, B. B. (2012). End of life: An overview. *Topics in Language Disorders, 32*(2), 111–118.

Toseland, R. W., Blanchard, C. G., & McCallion, P. (1995). A problem-solving intervention for caregivers of cancer patients. *Social Science & Medicine, 40*(4), 517–528.

Voepel-Lewis, T., Shayevitz, J. R., & Malviya, S. (1997). The FLACC: A behavioral scale for scoring postoperative pain in young children. *Pediatric Nursing, 23*(3), 293–297.

Volandes, A. E., Paasche-Orlow, M., Gillick, M. R., Cook, E. F., Shaykevich, S., Abbo, E. D., & Lehmann, L. (2008). Health literacy not race predicts end-of-life care preferences. *Journal of Palliative Medicine, 11*(5), 754–762. https://doi.org/10.1089/jpm.2007.0224

Wallace, G. (2013). Speech-language pathology: Enhancing quality of life for individuals approaching death. *Perspectives of the ASHA Special Interest Groups, 18*(3), 112–120. https://doi.org/10.1044/gero18.3.112

Williams, A. M. (2018). Education, training, and mentorship of caregivers of Canadians experiencing a life-limiting illness. *Journal of Palliative Medicine, 21*(S1), S45–S49. https://doi.org/10.1089/jpm.2017.0393

Wirz, S. L., Skinner, C., & Dean, E. (1990). *Revised Edinburgh Functional Communication Profile.* Communication Skill Builders.

Zarit, S., Reever, K., & Bach-Peterson, J. (1980). Relatives of the impaired elderly: Correlates of feelings of burden. *The Gerontologist, 20*(6), 649–655. https://doi.org/10.1093/geront/20.6.649

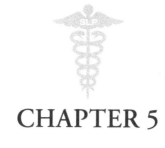

CHAPTER 5

Supporting Eating, Drinking, and Swallowing for Adults With Life-Limiting Conditions

Paula Leslie and Marnie Kershner

> *"The kind of changes that matter in the care of the chronically ill are usually not dramatic ones: they tend to be small changes in the perception of symptoms and in the tolerance of suffering. The space between a manageable distress and a defeating despair is often narrow."* —Kleinman, 1988, p. 249

INTRODUCTION

Evidence-based practice should remain at the forefront of our minds as we approach evaluation and treatment planning with each patient, regardless of their prognosis. Optimal clinical care integrates the best available evidence, informed clinician expertise, and informed patient goals and wishes (Sackett et al., 1996). As clinicians, we may be eager to initiate an intervention with a patient, but it is of the utmost importance that we start with the patient's priorities and readiness to participate. Patients may not be emotionally able to receive services, may not want services, or may not have the energy or stamina to participate. The patient's priorities are even more critical to ascertain in the inpatient setting or any situation in which the patient is not electing to come to us, but rather in which we arrive at their bedside or into their place of residence and invade their space.

Speech-language pathologists (SLPs) have worked with patients near the end of life (EoL) for as long as the profession has existed. What has changed is people's familiarity and understanding of EoL and dying. We often see terms such as "race for the cure" and "defeating cancer," which can minimize patients' experience of disease progression and enhance the view that illness and disease is to be conquered. Society, particularly in the West, has isolated the process of dying and the reality of death. High-profile athletes and celebrities are helping to open the dialogue by sharing their life-limiting diagnoses and their acceptance that not every disease can be overcome and that those who cannot "defeat" the illness have not failed in some way. Many newer clinicians have limited exposure to death and dying in their training. For example, a student in the second year of a health professions degree program once commented, "You are the first professor to tell us that some of our patients might die." This lack of training, coupled with sociocultural avoidance of death and dying, can leave clinicians uncertain or even fearful about how to support people who do not have an upward health trajectory and chance for recovery. SLPs have core skills in supporting these populations, given our skill set in counseling, communication, and familiarity with long-term health conditions that impact communication, cognition, eating, drinking, and swallowing (Xia, 2020).

Eating and drinking are fundamental to the human experience. Food and drink are deeply tied to culture, human social experience, and how humans show care for others from infancy and across the life span. Impairments that lead to difficulty with eating and/or drinking are not simply a matter of concern about the physiology of nutrition or hydration. They can cause significant distress to the person with such impairments, the family, and the professionals caring for that person. As Kleinman (1988) notes, small changes that ease function or reduce symptoms can keep someone out of despair. As you consider the many ways in which SLPs can support people with eating, drinking, and swallowing difficulties toward and at the EoL, consider, too, the appropriateness and timing of that help.

ESSENTIAL ROLES OF EATING, DRINKING, AND SWALLOWING (EDS)

Eating, drinking, and swallowing (EDS) processes perform two distinct and equally valuable roles for human beings. First, food

and drink are the essential fuel that serves the body's biological and mechanical functions. Such fuel enters the body system through two routes: enteral (into the intestinal system or gut) or nonenteral (into the bloodstream). The enteral route includes the typical oropharyngeal eating and drinking route and feeding tubes that may be placed in various parts of the gastrointestinal system. The nonenteral (or parenteral) route is used to administer medication into the bloodstream or intramuscularly. In addition, fluids and nutrition can be delivered into the bloodstream intravenously (IV). Food and fluid intake is required for the body whether we are healthy or living with a life-limiting condition. However, as people near the EoL, food and fluids may cause problems for body functions and can increase discomfort (Chahda et al., 2017).

The second role for EDS processes connects deeply to a person's identity, social connectedness, and relationships. If this role were not so significant, patients, families, and clinicians would experience much less angst when the EDS systems are impaired. Reflecting on what culture means to people nearly always includes food and drink, along with customs related to meals and even abstinence or fasting. The profound social and emotional importance of EDS can make the role of SLP feel very challenging. The psychosocial value of EDS is apparent when a recommendation for a restrictive diet is unacceptable to a patient and/or the patient's family because the recommendations related to EDS impact more than nutrition and hydration needs. It is critical that our recommendations account for both the patient's physiologic needs and the social role that food plays in people's lives.

We use the term "EDS impairments" as a deliberate move away from the narrow focus on the physiologic aspects of chewing and swallowing mechanics embedded in the terms "dysphagia" and "deglutition disorders." Much of SLPs' training in dysphagia focuses on the biomechanical model of swallowing; however, difficulties with eating for adequate nutrition and hydration may be located outside the tiny area of the pharynx that draws the SLP's laser-like gaze. Problems with vision, smell, taste, movement, cognition, and fatigue, for example, all impact the ability to obtain the nutrients that the body requires. Awareness of these factors is essential, as they directly inform assessment and treatment. Table 5–1 provides multiple examples of how EDS functions may be affected by a variety of clinical, physical, psychological, and social factors. We propose that the physiologic oropharyngeal "dysphagia" that has received so much historical focus be put in its place as a tiny component, given that there are so many other factors we can address and modify to support our patients and their families.

In this chapter, we will explore common conditions that may cause EDS impairments to provide the context in which these impairments may occur. As we approach care for patients nearing the EoL, special considerations will be addressed in a separate section for these conditions.

Table 5–1. Clinical and Psychosocial Factors to Consider in Assessment of Eating, Drinking, and Swallowing for Patients Nearing the End of Life

Domain	Example Considerations
Alertness and arousal	• Awake • Responsive to speech and voice • Able to follow one- or two-step commands
Primary diagnosis	• Is the primary diagnosis neurologic, oncologic, or other?
Secondary or other underlying diagnoses	• Does the patient have any other known diagnoses (e.g., diabetes, autism, kidney failure)?
Trajectory of dying (see Chapter 1)	• Does the patient have a terminal disease? Organ failure? Frailty? • Symptoms associated with active dying?
Sensory system considerations	• Vision • Hearing • Oral pain or sensitivity • Food texture or temperature issues
Physical considerations	• Gastrointestinal symptoms (e.g., constipation, diarrhea, nausea, discomfort) • Pain and level of pain control • Oral health • Positioning (e.g., able to sit independently in a chair)
Psychological considerations	• Fear or anxiety • Denial or acceptance of current health status • Documented diagnoses (e.g., depression)
Social considerations	• Setting (e.g., at home, in hospital) • Support (e.g., availability of family or other caregiver)

POPULATIONS AT RISK

EDS impairments are symptoms and not diseases themselves. Difficulty with EDS caused by other underlying diseases, disorders, or disruptions often follows a predictable path associated with the trajectory of the underlying etiology. Understanding the patient's causal diagnosis is essential to interpreting and predicting EDS status, course, and prognosis. Common groups of diseases and disorders in which EDS issues are likely to arise will be described below. This list is not exhaustive but illustrates the heterogeneity of EDS issues SLPs are likely to encounter with patients who are nearing the EoL.

The reported prevalence of EDS disorders for a given patient population varies widely in the literature (Rivelsrud et al., 2022). In part, these variances reflect differences in definition of EDS issues, assessment methods, the timing of swallow assessment, and sample size. Therefore, we will not review specific prevalence rates by diagnosis. Instead, the SLP should develop skills to identify the *possibility* of EDS impairments (or not) through careful chart review and patient interviews and use this personalized information to guide our clinical assessment. The goal is not to treat any patient as the textbook case for their given disease, but rather to treat the person in front of you. The aim in each clinical case is to sit down, be present with each patient, and determine evaluation and treatment plans that address *that* patient's needs.

Neurological Conditions

Progressive Neurologic Conditions

Common progressive neurological disorders associated with impairments in EDS include dementias (e.g., Alzheimer type, vascular, frontotemporal, and Lewy body), amyotrophic lateral sclerosis (ALS), Parkinson's disease, multiple sclerosis (MS), muscular dystrophies (e.g., Duchenne muscular dystrophy), and Huntington's disease. Early in the disease course, the SLP may focus on education, counseling, and skills maintenance, and SLP interventions must evolve as the patient's EDS abilities change. As EDS skills gradually decline, mealtime modifications and limitations increase and the focus may be to reduce dysphagia-related illness, reduce frequency of uncomfortable coughing, and/or to provide comfort-focused strategies. Ideally, SLPs work with patients over time, allowing for multiple points of informed decision making between the patient, their family, and their medical team regarding EDS management.

Acute Injury

Acute neurological insults to the brain, such as stroke or traumatic brain injury, pose the most significant risks at the time of the event. With timely and appropriate medical care, such injuries tend not to be life limiting due to the brain's incredible plasticity. EDS impairments following stroke and traumatic brain injury typically improve with time. However, for some, the nature and scope of the insult from an acute event can start a cascade of clinical complications that lead to poor outcomes. In these situations, patients' health status may decline quite quickly. Progressive neurological disorders typically afford time for significant counseling, adjustment, and gradual adjustments to plans. In contrast, acute neurological insults that are life limiting in nature rarely allow this. In some health care systems, the SLP is consulted as a matter of routine to clear a patient for eating and drinking at the time of admission after a stroke or brain injury. In cases where the SLP is involved with a patient post stroke, the SLP should review the medical status thoroughly and be aware that EDS disorders may be one of many comorbidities, ultimately leading to a rapid trajectory toward the EoL.

Oncological Conditions

The links between EDS impairments and cancer are both direct and indirect. Direct EDS impairments may occur due to changes in structure and function of the chewing and swallowing mechanism, such as surgical removal of structures of the head and neck (e.g., tongue, larynx, velum, or tonsillar pillars) or physiologic changes in tissue associated with radiation therapy in the head and neck region. Indirect EDS impairments are associated with cancer treatments and are not limited to head and neck cancers. Moving down the digestive tract, esophageal, stomach, and bowel/colon cancers each have clear physical impacts on EDS functioning. Cancers can significantly diminish overall functional status, which in and of itself places patients at risk for EDS impairments. EDS function may serve as a barometer of the body's overall level of functioning and, as metabolic demands associated with cancer increase, these demands may compound EDS impairments and act as another barrier to achieving adequate nutrition and hydration.

Chemotherapy

Chemotherapy is the use of chemical agents designed to kill rapidly replicating cancer cells. Chemotherapy impacts other rapidly replicating cells such as the epithelial lining of the mouth and gastrointestinal system. Common acute impacts of chemotherapy for any form of cancer include nausea, vomiting, fatigue, constipation and/or diarrhea, loss of appetite, mouth sores, and altered taste sensation, any of which may impact EDS processes. Chemotherapies suppress immune system func-

tion and can place patients at increased risk for infection and adverse outcomes if EDS impairments are present.

Longer-term impacts of chemotherapy, which can lead to EDS impairments, include altered taste sensation, xerostomia (dry mouth), and dental and oral health issues. Cardiac and pulmonary complications can raise the risk of adverse outcomes when EDS impairments are present. The increased metabolic needs associated with cancers can exacerbate barriers to adequate nutrition resulting from EDS impairments. This, in turn, can lead to a negative feedback loop, as depicted in Figure 5–1. For example, a patient with dysphagia and cancer may struggle to maintain adequate nutrition and hydration due to the impact of treatment side effects and decreased mealtime efficiency, which adds to the nutrition/hydration deficit already present due to the

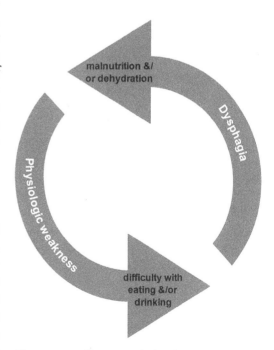

Figure 5–1. The association between decline in eating, drinking, and swallowing function and malnutrition that yields increased difficulties with oral intake.

cancer. The decline of the patient's nutrition/hydration status then exacerbates dysphagia in a continuous cycle of decline.

Radiation Therapy

Radiation can impact EDS very close to the time of radiation treatment (acutely) and in the long term (chronically). Acute radiation impacts may include xerostomia, mucositis, and fatigue. Late effects of radiation may include xerostomia, thick secretions, dental issues, reduced jaw range of motion (trismus), and pain with swallowing (odynophagia). For patients who avoid swallowing due to these side effects, disuse atrophy can further exacerbate EDS impairments.

Combined Therapies

Surgery, radiation therapy, and chemotherapy are often combined or offered in sequence over time. Combined therapies, particularly the combination of radiation and chemotherapy, can compound the side effects of these treatments. For example, patients with head and neck cancer who receive combined radiation and chemotherapy have a greater likelihood of swallowing impairment than those who receive one form of treatment in isolation (Lazarus, 2009). A key takeaway is that the impacts of cancer and its treatments can lead to numerous EDS impairments and that EDS impairments are likely to change in association with treatment regimens and over the course of disease progression (American Society of Clinical Oncology, 2019; Barbon et al., 2017).

Patients With Multiple Medical Conditions

Patients with multiple chronic medical conditions are at greater risk for developing EDS impairments and adverse outcomes (including death) due to compounding diagnoses (Langmore et al., 1998; Nativ-Zeltzer et al., 2022). Examples of common chronic medical conditions include hypertension, diabetes, chronic obstructive pulmonary disease (COPD), asthma, chronic kidney disease, and heart disease. Patients may have more than one chronic disease or may experience acute or progressive illness(es) in addition to existing chronic illness.

As noted earlier, EDS impairments are a symptom or outcome of underlying disorders or disruptions and may reflect overall systemic function. If you think of the body as a machine, such as a car, one or two systems can stop working, and the car will still run. However, there will be a point when the cumulative system failures are too much and the car will not be able to run. That final "system failure" for humans may be a new EDS impairment. As we review our patients' medical histories, it is helpful to keep this concept in mind and consider the individual's total disease burden and functional reserve.

NATURE OF EATING, DRINKING, AND SWALLOWING CONCERNS FOR PEOPLE NEAR THE END OF LIFE

EDS impairments affect people near the EoL in the same ways that they might affect any of us—mealtimes are disrupted, favorite foods are restricted or prohibited, the person may experience fear or guilt about eating or not eating meals prepared for them, and those around them may feel guilty about eating freely. In all circumstances, the SLP must consider the mechanical and psychosocial aspects of EDS function and how these interact. When someone's ability to participate in their culture changes, that impacts them socially and emotionally. When someone's physical abilities change, that impacts them psychologically, socially, and emotionally. When someone's cognitive status is altered, this, too, has an emotional impact. Thus hearing, acknowledging, and supporting patient emotions is a fundamental skill for clinicians (Ambuel, 2004).

Cultural Impacts

Humans need three things in the biomechanical model of health: (a) oxygen, (b) fuel, and (c) an oxygen/fuel processing system. Notably, we choose what, where, and with whom only with fuel. Eating, drinking, swallowing, and feeding are individual acts signaling our values, identity, and cultural alignment. All cultures use food, fasting (deliberate absence of food), and specific foods to mark celebrations, sadness, transitions, and milestones. We all have foods that, to us, are a delight; to others, the same foods would be the last thing they want to see on a plate. For example, in a British grocery store magazine, a love letter is written to peanut butter and the comfort it brings:

> *"The feeling was always the same: smooth (never crunchy—but that is a debate for another day), soothing comfort."*—Tandoh, 2021, p. 17

In this simple example, we see a clear preference for what is considered the correct type of peanut butter. It is important to note that while some adore peanut butter and find it comforting, many people find the same foodstuff revolting.

Food and drink, and abstinence from them, are wired into us from an early age. Specific foods, tastes, and smells are deeply linked to memory and can transport us to another time and place. A person's culture comprises years of experiences and connections to people and places. Cultural identity transcends time

and geography. Even the slightest change in preparation, presentation, setting, or social context may disrupt the person's experience, with profound consequences (Dalton et al., 2022). We only need to reflect on how we prepare a family dish or the expectation that celebratory meal items will appear in a particular form (and not as a giant smoothie) to appreciate that eating and drinking, and food and drink, are far more than nutritional fuel for a machine.

Physical Considerations

From a physiologic perspective, food and fluid intake are as essential to life as oxygen. The process of eating and drinking is a complex, beautifully coordinated dance of cognitive processes, muscle movements, breath holding, and valve sequencing. When ancestral humans moved to vertical motion and started talking, some design flaws emerged as the tiny tube containing the airway entrance and the food pipe aligned. This alignment, which leaves open a connection between the respiratory and digestive systems, spells disaster if the two pathways do not separate as they are supposed to. Failure can only be averted by this amazing physiological choreography that shuts the entrance to the airway, pulls the larynx up, opens a set of valves, and propels food from the mouth to the esophagus in less than a second (Martin et al., 1994). This highly coordinated sequence is followed immediately by the respiratory system opening again so we can breathe, which is always our primary biologic driver.

Part of many disease processes and decline toward the EoL is an expected reduction of food and fluid intake. As intake falls, it is common for people nearing the EoL to experience dehydration, loss of muscle mass, weight loss, and weakness. Lack of protein and energy intake is the most common type of malnutrition in developed countries and leads to weight loss. Individuals who have EDS dysfunction(s) are at risk for protein/energy malnutrition (Veldee & Peth, 1992). As nutritional intake decreases, other physical and behavioral changes occur such as skin breakdown (Banks et al., 2010), fatigue, diminished attention and memory (Schuetz et al., 2021), and heightened risk of infection (Fan et al., 2022). In turn, the muscles are weakened, which contributes to further difficulty with EDS functions in an ongoing cycle of functional decline (see Figure 5–1).

Adequate hydration is necessary for cellular homeostasis and life. From a body-systems perspective, hydration is essential in balancing blood volume, which impacts blood pressure and heart rate, kidney function (Popkin et al., 2010), and bowel function. The consequences of dehydration include increased blood pressure, headache, oral dryness and discomfort, constipation, falls, kidney impairment, deep vein thrombosis, hospitalization rate, and increased length of hospital stay. Even mild dehydration can negatively impact cognitive functioning, mood, and level of arousal. For patients with underlying health conditions, dehydration can exacerbate these conditions (McCotter et al., 2016; Oates & Price, 2017; Popkin et al., 2010). Older adults may have lower physiological resilience to dehydration, making them more susceptible to constipation (Morley, 2015). As patients near the EoL, maintaining adequate hydration may be complicated by the reduced opportunity for fluid intake (e.g., an individual who has limited mobility and relies on others for food and drink), medications impacting hydration either directly (e.g., diuretics) or indirectly (e.g., chemotherapeutics), incontinence (which may lead to avoidance of fluid intake), and/or EDS impairments (Bunn et al., 2015; McCotter et al., 2016; Popkin et al., 2010).

Constipation is a common side effect of pain medications, particularly opioids, which can lead to nausea, discomfort, and the need for additional interventions, so maintaining hydration is often a specific goal that accompanies the introduction of pain medications in palliative and hospice care. The focus on oral intake, along with the cascade of side effects associated with nutrition and hydration issues, is unwelcome for the person near the EoL and often add to the overall illness burden.

Cognitive Considerations

Cognitive impairments may be a source of EDS impairment, may exacerbate EDS impairments, or may be negatively affected by EDS impairments themselves. Cognition plays an essential role in eating and drinking, including in the acts leading up to a snack or meal. Leopold and Kagel (1997) proposed a preoral phase emphasizing the role of stimuli such as the smells of food, the sounds of dishes, and food preparation that each provide important subconscious cognitive clues and inform the phases to follow (e.g., inducing salivation and early activation of neural circuits involved in swallowing). Cognitive processes such as arousal, motivation, planning, initiation, attention, and safety awareness allow us to integrate neurological, motor, and sensory systems to successfully manipulate and swallow a bolus. EDS impairments affecting nutrition or hydration can contribute to changes in cognition.

Medication and Pain Management Considerations

Many life-limiting conditions require palliative medication to manage symptoms and side effects of other treatments. The side effects of such medicines include sedation, xerostomia, and cognitive changes such as delirium. SLPs do not prescribe medication, but knowledge of types of medications and their impacts is vital to our understanding of patient care and to meaningful treatment planning (Lawton, 2022). Disease processes affect eating, drinking, and swallowing, and these impacts may also be compounded by medications used to treat the disease or those used for symptom management. The gastrointestinal tract is one long tube, and problems at any point along it will impact both upstream and downstream function. For example, a frequent side effect and drawback of many pain relief medicines is constipation (Dzierzanowski & Mercadante, 2022), which may seem a long way from oropharyngeal function, but gastrointestinal discomfort, bloating, and other symptoms negatively impact appetite.

In another vicious cycle, impairments to the EDS processes may limit the types of medications a person can use without requiring skilled nursing care. Pharmacological treatments can depress the body's defense systems and increase risk for opportunistic infections, such as oral thrush. Finally, the psychological importance of mealtimes may also be affected if a person's ability to participate in meals is limited by sedation, endurance, oral discomfort, or other difficulties with oral intake.

Fatigue Considerations

Fatigue is a frequent symptom of underlying disease progression, medical treatments, and the burden of chronic illness. Malnutrition and dehydration increase fatigue and decrease the desire to eat. SLPs need to understand that a patient's decreasing interest and motivation to eat is an expected part of the trajectory toward death. Strategies such as frequent small meals and paced eating may help.

One way to consider pacing is proposed by Miserandino (2003), who described the finite energy available to people with chronic disease represented by a certain number of spoons available for use in a day. In the "spoon theory," each task uses up one or more spoons and the individual with chronic disease must decide how best to distribute their spoons each day. This requires careful planning for energy use and includes tasks that healthy people may not consider, such as the demands of taking a shower, getting dressed, and visiting with a neighbor. For those near the EoL, eating and drinking can consume many spoons because meal preparation and consumption take time, energy, and care. For some patients with chronic disease, it is a relief to begin supplemental nutrition through high-energy drinks or foods or to initiate artificially administered hydration and nutrition, such as nasogastric tube feeding. For others, the pleasure of oral eating, the taste and texture of food and drink, and the social aspects of sharing a meal are essential to quality of life and they will reserve "spoons" for this pleasure.

IMPACT OF EATING, DRINKING, AND SWALLOWING IMPAIRMENTS ON FAMILY AND SUPPORT NETWORKS

When EDS functions are impacted by disease, the consequences are felt by the patient and those in their close networks, especially family (Shune et al., 2022). Assessments and treatment plans for dysphagia often focus on the patient, but most people eat and drink with others in a shared mealtime and social context. The patient may be the main food preparer for a family and not just a participant or recipient of meals. Consequences of impaired EDS can include increased duration of meals, difficulty with certain foods, coughing or choking, and lack of interest in eating. These consequences impact all persons involved in the patient's mealtimes. Family celebrations, religious and spiritual events, life transitions, and cultural engagement may all be affected for the patient and those in their social circles (Leslie & Broll, 2022; Leslie et al., 2021; Padilla et al., 2019; Shune et al., 2022).

SLPs need to be aware of and sensitive to the impact of illness and care among family and other personal caregivers. Not all family members or friends of a patient will be comfortable discussing issues with members of the health care team, particularly in front of the patient. Conversely, in some situations, the patient, even when they have full capacity, is not the locus of the decision-making process (Childers, 2019; Kleinman, 1988). Family members face the trials of trying to do their best for the person near the EoL while attempting to maintain the life they know, such as holding on to the social importance of certain foods and eating rituals (Wallin et al., 2014).

For most families dealing with EoL care, there is a great deal of physical and psychological burden (Ellis, 2018). Clinicians must be mindful not to ask family members to do more than they can manage and to acknowledge that our involvement with families is relatively fleeting. For example, our thoughtful recommendation to have smaller and more frequent meals may increase a perceived burden of food preparation. It is essential that recommendations are practical and responsive to the full social context of care. Caregivers should be invited to discuss recommendations, to ask questions, and to work alongside the SLP to develop and implement EDS strategies.

EVALUATION OF EATING, DRINKING, AND SWALLOWING DIFFICULTIES FOR PEOPLE NEAR THE END OF LIFE

Before we rush to consider clinical and instrumental assessments, we should discuss the possible costs, benefits, and outcomes with the patient, family, and other health care team members (Lawton, 2022; see also Chapter 3). In this context, "costs" does not necessarily refer to financial costs, but rather to broad consideration of negative outcomes such as harms or suffering that may be associated with a given course of action. We, as clinicians, know the likely issues and outcomes. An important precept in health care is to do tests only if the results will contribute to feasible and valuable interventions. Discussing the costs, benefits, and outcomes of clinical assessments allows the patient and their family to reflect on why a test might be helpful or not and to participate in shared decision making. Patients might decide not to proceed with an assessment because the implications of findings would not change their desired plan of care or possible interventions would be unacceptable. This approach results in treatment plans that align with the patient's preferences and may prove less burdensome for the patient. When clinicians focus on the patient's goals and preferences, both assessment and treatment planning will be more efficient.

When shared decision making is implemented, it is more likely that patients and their caregivers will be comfortable with the recommendations and more invested in the outcomes. The patient (and/or caregiver) and clinician will be much better aligned concerning acceptable outcomes and recommendations, thus limiting any sense of adversarial "them" and "us."

In all clinical relationships, the SLP needs to plan for discharge from the outset of each encounter because our involvement is time limited. Discharge is a topic that gets less attention than assessment and intervention in clinical training. However, it is essential to discuss discharge goals to manage expectations and lessen patient distress, particularly in palliative care (Roe & Leslie, 2010).

Establishing Patient and Caregiver Understanding of Their Status

We must share information to ensure patients and families can make informed decisions. This sharing is a two-way cyclical process and is really what the "counseling" process means in our scope of practice (Lawton, 2022). Clinicians bring information in a generalized form about EDS conditions and possible outcomes. Patients and families bring specific information about personal experiences and impacts. The SLP and the family work through an interative process, each educating the other to understand the situation. The clinician's responsibility is to engage the patient and their family in meaningful conversation and empower them to ask questions they did not know they needed to ask. This clear understanding will enable the clinician to offer the most tailored and specific information for that patient and to engage in a process of shared decision making (see also Chapter 3).

Clinicians build expertise and knowledge through training and clinical experience. Clinicians can fall into the trap of presuming knowledge or underappreciating the impact of EDS and health issues on the patient or family for whom all symptoms, assessments, and interventions are new (Dickens et al., 2013; Hayes & Bajzek, 2008). The SLP's familiarity with EDS issues may make us blind to the patient's and family's experience. In the context of EoL care, the assumptions the SLP brings to a clinical relationship can combine poorly with a lack of exposure and comfort with discussing EoL issues. Thus, meaningful conversations may be difficult to initiate. Our role as experienced clinicians is to set up the environment so that patients and families feel more comfortable engaging in discussions. Using our professional skills in effective communication, we can optimize the exchange of information. We can ensure understanding by asking the patient or family members to explain their understanding, issues, and rationales to us and, where needed we can provide missing information sensitively to help educate the patient, other members of their family, and the care team. The patient should be consulted about their preference for family members and other support caregivers in these discussions. Essential concepts to have effective discussions include:

- Set up the discussions in advance.
- Establish a level of health literacy (which is not the same as education).
- Consider individual culture and comfort with discussing health issues.
- Establish what people know before offering advice.
- Ask the patient for their permission to discuss matters.
- Communicate clearly and avoid use of medical or clinical jargon.

There are several valuable guides designed for health professionals to support effective communication and counseling strategies. One example is the SPIKES protocol, which guides the clinician through practical issues such as ensuring privacy and quiet, establishing the patient's awareness and knowledge, and strategies for sharing clinical information and for collaborating with the patient to establish a plan (Baile et al., 2000). The Explanatory Model advises we ask "what," "why," "how," and "who" questions to help bridge the gap between the clinician's perspectives and those of the patient and family (Kleinman et al., 1978). Example questions include "What do you think might be causing this problem?" or "How do you think we could best help you?" Effective counseling approaches are critical for all clinicians who aim to meet the needs of the patient and family through cultural humility, responsiveness, and respect.

Context

The location in which the person receives our care matters. Acute hospitals differ from rehabilitation settings, and inpatients face different challenges to outpatients. Rarely are clinicians lucky enough to support patients as they move across these health care settings. Excellent communication between clinicians across settings and disciplines is necessary for continuity of services and for patients to experience good care. The exchange of information across settings can be challenging in a fractured system and with data-sharing restrictions. Communication across settings can be further limited by the overuse of medical jargon, which is confusing for patients, may not be consistent across professionals, and may vary from one setting or institution to another. Continuity of care is essential for those with life-limiting conditions and for the EoL. The requirement for patients to continue endless repetition of their condition, symptoms, medications, interventions, and medical history compounds the fatigue patients feel, which we could effectively address if we communicated better as clinicians. Effective and efficient information exchange between all stakeholders limits mistakes, optimizes care, and reduces the burden on the patient and the patient's family.

Inpatient Contexts

Within an inpatient context, such as acute care, clinicians are often managing patients with a severe critical injury or a severe decline in health status from a primary illness. When patients are admitted with pneumonia, develop pneumonia, or have difficulty with oral intake, it is common practice to consult with SLP services. Clinicians should expect to provide families with information and clear recommendations as to options and next steps. The acute nature of these events or rapid decline often means that families have

little time for emotional adjustment to the situation. The rapidity of clinical decline and onset of complications requires clinicians to engage in discussions about goals of care with little chance to develop a clinical relationship. The pace of the acute care setting places an additional responsibility on clinicians to present each option, discuss the costs and benefits of the options available, and engage in shared decision making with the patient and family. This includes providing families with alternatives to feeding tube placements, such as hand feeding or other comfort care measures.

Outpatient Clinic Contexts

The person living at home and coming in as an outpatient may bring motivation and expectation to an appointment. They have made an effort and seek clinical care. Patients and family members may look forward to a clinic appointment and opportunity to connect with a clinician with whom they have formed a bond. However, it is equally likely that patients experience fatigue and burden associated with the effort of preparation, travel, transport, and wait times associated with outpatient visits. As people near the EoL, caregivers and patients may find outpatient visits overly burdensome. Clinicians should be aware that patients may not want to share that they are not coping well at home.

Home Visits

Home visits reduce the burden on patients and caregivers and give the clinician a better sense of the patient's environment, support mechanisms, and restrictions. Home visits allow the SLP to identify the availability of food and drink, who is involved in meal preparation, availability of seating, and any specialized equipment. Toward the EoL, the demands are often more significant on the patient and on the family's time, and resources may be stretched thin. Improving our situational awareness allows us to be more in tune with what the patient and family need and can manage (Roe & Leslie, 2010; Xia, 2020). If possible, home visits should be negotiated and conducted in the context of an interprofessional team.

Appetite

An essential role for the SLP is to identify modifiable factors that can reduce or relieve symptoms or suffering for patients who are nearing the EoL. Appetite is closely associated with the pleasure of eating and drinking and can be negatively impacted by various easily modifiable factors (Kershner & Askren, 2022). Unfortunately, these factors are often overlooked as a patient's medical status becomes increasingly complex and precarious. Potential barriers to appetite and recommended interventions to overcome these barriers are shown in Table 5–2.

Not all factors that contribute to lack of appetite can be modified for a given patient, but often one or more modifications can be made with impact on the patient's experience with EDS and associated decrease in burden for caregivers. Therefore, the goal is not to eliminate every factor but to identify which factors can be addressed to optimize each patient's appetite.

INTERVENTION PLANS FOR EATING, DRINKING, AND SWALLOWING DIFFICULTIES FOR PEOPLE NEAR THE END OF LIFE

Many traditional management strategies for EDS impairments require careful consideration for patients nearing the EoL (and across

Table 5–2. Potential Barriers to Patient Appetite and Interventions to Reduce Impact on Appetite

Potential Barrier to Appetite	Possible Intervention
Drug-induced alteration in taste (dysgeusia)	• Medication review
Xerostomia	• Medication review • Over-the-counter oral moisturizer spray or liquid • Excellent oral care • Ice chips, popsicles • Hard candy, if oral control allows
Fear of incontinence	• Toileting schedule
Poor positioning with meals	• Transfer from bed to a chair for meals
Foul odors associated with wounds or toileting	• Schedule nursing care at different times from meals
Feelings of isolation or loneliness	• Facilitate company for meals (in-person or virtually)
Mismatch between home and hospital routines	• Match meal times with home routines as much as possible • Encourage family to bring in preferred foods and drinks from home

other patient groups). For example, we have little evidence that modifying food or liquid textures helps with long-term outcomes (Beck et al., 2018; Wu et al., 2020). Instead, the evidence indicates that this practice results in reduced consumption of food and drink, fear, embarrassment, loss of autonomy, and withdrawal from social activities (Lazenby-Paterson, 2020; Lippert et al., 2019; Steele et al., 2021; Wang et al., 2016). Modifying textures is time-consuming and costly, needs special equipment and commercial thickeners, and can alter taste and texture of food in negative ways. Additional burden of special food preparation may inadvertently separate the patient from regular family mealtimes (McCurtin et al., 2018). Such isolation is not desirable as patients' health status declines and is closely associated with depression.

Patients and families often express preference for particular foods that may be associated with personal favorites, family or cultural traditions, or special significance. In discussions about favored foods, we must explore how these preferences align with the SLP's recommendations and recognize that the SLP's preferences have little relevance for the patient who is nearing the EoL.

To serve patients with life-limiting conditions, it is essential that the SLP be well acquainted with the trajectory of disease before discussing options for food and fluid intake with patients and their families (see also Chapter 1). For example, early in the course of head and neck cancer, tube feeding is the standard of care (Kristensen et al., 2020) and there are specific situations such as short-term supplementation of nutrition and hydration that offer a benefit to patients. Examples include preparation for surgery or radiation therapy (Kristensen et al., 2020) or during acute illness or short-term relief from fatigue (Carter, 2020). On the other hand, tube feeding is contraindicated as patients

enter the final stages of disease. Lack of appetite (anorexia), muscle wasting (cachexia), and slowed metabolism are expected as people near death. During this stage, as metabolic function diminishes, people do not experience hunger and thirst in the same way as they did when healthy. Pushing food and fluid may increase discomfort and burden for the patient. It is well understood that the potential harms of tube feeding outweigh the benefits for patients with advanced dementia who may experience increased pain, risk of infection and aspiration, and use of restraints associated with tube feeding with no expected increase in life expectancy or other clinical benefits (Carter, 2020; Flaschner & Katz, 2015; Goldberg & Altman, 2014; Hallenbeck, 2015; McCann et al., 1994). Thus, evaluation of costs and benefits associated with oral intake and with artificially administered food and fluid is highly relevant to patient and family decisions at each stage of disease progression.

Intervention plans should account for the impact of medication on EDS and meal participation (see Chapter 1). Potential medication side effects that may impact EDS include nausea (e.g., antibiotics, antidepressants, chemotherapy drugs), reduced appetite (e.g., stimulants), xerostomia (a widespread side effect of many drug types), reduced level of arousal/sedation (e.g., antiepileptics, benzodiazepines, antipsychotics, antidepressants), and gastroesophageal reflux (e.g., anticholinergics; Lawton et al., 2022).

If medication intake is a goal of EDS-related intervention, the SLP should be aware of or should verify the impact of crushing medication for ease of intake. For example, many patients enrolled in hospice care receive extended-release morphine (or other opioids). Tablets and capsules designed for slow release of morphine over 8 to 12 hours, if crushed or dissolved in liquid, will deliver a very large and potentially dangerous dose of morphine.

Specialized Knowledge and Professional Competence

It is rare that graduate education in speech-language pathology includes coverage of pharmacologic agents, their classifications, effects, and side effects. Similarly, most of the evidence associated with the costs and benefits of oral intake, careful hand feeding, and artificially administered food and fluids through various forms of tube feeding is in the medical literature, not the speech-language pathology literature. As in every area of practice, it is the SLPs' responsibility to grow their knowledge base through continued reading and professional development. Professional competence also requires recognition of "knowing what you don't know," which includes the responsibility for consultation with members of the care team and/or referral to other experts (Lawton et al., 2022). As SLPs establish their role as a member of a hospice or palliative care team, consultation and collaboration are essential to ensure accurate counseling and reasonable recommendations and to uphold the goals of palliative care that balance patients' quality of life with comfort and safety for them and support for their caregivers.

DOCUMENTATION AND USE OF LANGUAGE

The words we use to describe EDS impairments influence our practice, how other professionals interpret our assessment and recommendations and, most importantly, the patient experience. Therefore, we urge you to consider phrasing and terminology when speaking to patients, their families, and others on their care team, as well as in your documentation. For example, rather than documenting

a patient's performance as "risky" or "unsafe," instead concretely describe what was observed along with the potential consequences. A sample clinical note:

> During the instrumental examination [VFSS or FEES], Mx. Smith swallowed X and Y without difficulty, but with Z [what happened]. This could cause Mx. Smith to [describe the potential consequence]. We discussed these findings with Mx. Smith, who expressed their understanding by explaining back to us "[what Mx. Smith said]" and that their preference is to [what Mx. Smith said].

Similarly, rather than referring to a patient who requires assistance with self-feeding as "a feeder" (in line with the language we would use to describe farm animals), consider person-first language such as "patient requires assistance with self-feeding."

Importance of Addressing Communication and Cognition With Eating, Drinking, and Swallowing Intervention

Knowledge of a patient's cognitive/communication status is essential to developing an EDS plan of care. This knowledge shapes how we present information to patients and informs our recommendations. Our recommendations must match patients' informed goals, wishes, abilities, and resources. A complex swallow maneuver, for example, is an inappropriate recommendation for a patient who cannot reliably follow two-step commands. Modifications such as using smaller spoons or a flow-control cup may be more appropriate interventions for patients struggling to recall new information rather than instructing them to take smaller bites and sips. A self-advocacy goal is inappropriate for a patient who does not have insight into their EDS impairments. For a patient whose cognitive deficits are driving their EDS issues, those cognitive skills may be more appropriate targets to support or augment than the EDS acts themselves. For example, reducing environmental distractions during meals is preferable to setting goals to reduce aspiration risk or swallow function for a patient nearing the EoL. As with everything we do, we must consider the whole patient.

Focus on Functional Goals

Historically, speech-language pathology has been considered a rehabilitation profession; our work aims to improve function. The range of improvement is broad and can encompass physical changes, knowledge and use of compensatory strategies, and enhanced patient and/or caregiver participation in education. For example, in the acute care setting, we may work to improve patient understanding and implementation of good oral hygiene practices. In the home setting, we may work with patients to identify environmental modifications that support safety and comfort during meals, such as sitting upright in their wheelchair or at the kitchen table. SLPs can also support people to maintain function, slow the impact of decline, and maximize quality of life. These are appropriate goals, and in systems where payment is required for health care, such interventions are covered by insurance if defined appropriately (American Speech-Language-Hearing Association [ASHA], n.d.-a). Patient and caregiver education is also an appropriate goal, particularly if we can show how this education directly impacts function. Examples of reimbursable goals are provided in Table 5–3 (see also Chapter 2).

Functional goals are, by definition, highly individualized. When the clinician is with an individual, the focus should be entirely on the person in front of them, and not on what we think we know or bring from some textbook read in school (including this one)! Good general texts can guide the novice clinician to think about goals (e.g., Gozdziewski et al., 2019). However, the literature often focuses heavily on physiology rather than the psychological and social aspects of EDS issues that must be considered near the EoL.

Although professional knowledge and skill in dysphagia and processes of EDS are essential, it is also critical that the SLP develop comfort with death, dying, and EoL care. Our goal is to help patients and families feel more at ease or at least not to add to their distress because of our discomfort with talking about death and dying. Clinicians must remain alert to how personal discomfort is conveyed through nonverbal cues and actions and how we discuss clinical information and recommendations. Societal avoidance of death and dying is pervasive in many western cultures; clinicians can counter this through exposure to the perspectives of those who are dying, available in many firsthand accounts that explore existential crises alongside finding peace and satisfaction of a life well lived (e.g., Albom, 2007; Yedida & MacGregor, 2001). Please see Appendix C for additional resources.

There is not, nor should there be, a standard set of strategies for addressing EDS impairments when the prognosis is poor. As you develop a treatment plan, goals should focus on living well. Example questions to identify specific goals for a given patient might be "How can we help you live well?" or "What makes you happy?" (Ambuel, 2016). Explore with the patient and family if there are favorite foods the patient would like to eat but has previously avoided to uphold healthy eating or other dietary restrictions. Although the

Table 5–3. Sample Reimbursable Goals Related to Eating, Drinking, Swallowing, and Dysphagia Management for Patients Nearing the End of Life

Reduction of symptom burden goals	• Patient will demonstrate use of compensatory swallowing strategies with minimal verbal prompts with 100% accuracy over four consecutive sessions to decrease discomfort of coughing and risk of aspiration
	• Patient will attend to the feeding task using compensatory strategies for a minimum of 20 minutes at mealtimes to increase caloric intake
	• Patient will initiate self-feeding using visual cues in seven of 10 opportunities to increase caloric intake
	• Patient will initiate a drink to cleanse the oral cavity after every two bites of food to increase residue clearance in 90% of tracked opportunities
	• The patient will consume one-third cup ice chips (½″ pieces or smaller) within 30 minutes without overt signs of aspiration in 70% of trials for pleasure and comfort
Caregiver/ family training goals	• Caregiver will demonstrate appropriate cleaning and maintenance of patient's oral cavity, with minimal clinician cues, over three consecutive sessions, to decrease the patient's risk of aspiration pneumonia, and increase patient comfort
	• Caregiver will demonstrate safe suctioning of the patient's oral cavity following mealtime with minimal clinician cues, over two consecutive sessions, to decrease the patient's risk of aspiration pneumonia and increase patient comfort
	• Caregiver will demonstrate careful hand-feeding procedures with minimal clinician cues, over two consecutive sessions, to decrease the patient's risk of aspiration pneumonia and increase patient comfort
	• Caregiver will describe the differences between choking and aspiration events using teach-back with 90% accuracy
	• Caregiver will explain the difference between the need to eat and drink for pleasure and the goals of nutrition maintenance through teach-back with 90% accuracy
Physiologic goals	• The patient will complete 15 repetitions of stretching and range-of-motion exercises 2–3 times per day given moderate verbal cues to preserve adequate jaw opening for eating and drinking

patient and family do not require permission to eat high-calorie (high-fat, high-sugar, high-salt) foods, some patients will benefit when a health care professional specifically says "It's OK to eat" whatever foods they have identified as desirable.

Broad topics the SLP should include in a checklist for all patients with a terminal illness or those nearing the EoL include secretion management, oral hygiene, oral comfort, ways to reduce distressing symptoms during eating such as excessive coughing or shortness of breath, patient and family education, and self-advocacy.

Family and Caregiver Involvement in the Intervention Plan

A significant component of our work with patients nearing the EoL is family and caregiver education with focus on support related to EDS processes, difficulties observed and expected, and interventions. Sometimes interventions are simple ideas or strategies to optimize eating and drinking, and SLPs bring a wealth of knowledge and solutions from working with many patient populations. Integration of family members and other caregivers is important for all parties because eating, drinking, preparing food, and feeding are intimate acts. Careful hand feeding is an act of service and helps families to feel they are doing something worthwhile in a context that often limits their sense of control and ability to contribute.

Understanding the dying process and the physical body's needs is critical to supporting both the patient and those close to them (Chahda et al., 2017; Roe & George, 2016). Family members are at risk of feeling they must do something, which often includes a desire to feed the patient because food and drink are so integral to our lives and social systems of nurture and care. It can be a relief to patients and caregivers when goals of care shift from measures of calorie intake to eating and drinking for pleasure alone. When food and fluid intake no longer contribute to the patient's well-being, SLPs can support caregivers through education and encourage substitute activities that maintain the caring relationship. One example is oral care, which is also an intimate act between two people. The physiological and psychological importance of oral care should be reflected in goals included in every care plan (NHS Ayrshire & Arran, 2017; McCann et al., 1994). Oral care enables family members to transfer the care they associate with providing food and drink to a more appropriate undertaking that contributes to the patient's comfort and well-being.

For all our carefully reasoned recommendations and ideas for family involvement, we must maintain an awareness of any plan's burden on them. The practicalities of who

is available, who is the decision maker, how comfortable they are with helping, and to what level they wish to be involved all need to be addressed sensitively. People may initially feel uncomfortable admitting that they will struggle, that they are scared, and that they do not have the capacity to offer resources given the broad array of care needs, grief, and other responsibilities they may be managing. Family food practices and relationships are not always about selfless care. They may raise tensions in families as members strive for their voices to be heard, bring the reality of death closer, and remind people of things that are now being lost (Ellis, 2018). Our broad skills as professionals with experience and capacity to support and counsel scared and vulnerable people in times of stress and uncertainty are well suited to offer thoughtful and empathetic care for patients and their families.

Traditional Intervention

Once all the factors above have been considered, we may reflect on traditional SLP approaches to manage EDS difficulties and associated symptoms:

- modification (e.g., diet consistency);
- compensation (e.g., changing the environment); and
- rehabilitation (e.g., muscle relearning).

For people with life-limiting conditions, the rehabilitation goals of recovery toward baseline is usually the least likely approach. More appropriate goals will focus on modification and compensation to maintain function for as long as possible, reduce the rate of decline, and support patients and families as they cope with ongoing decline in function.

Nasogastric tubes are sometimes introduced in the acute care setting when there are significant barriers to initiating or maintaining an oral diet. The decision to use short-term alternative means of nutrition and hydration is often driven by multiple factors that extend beyond the integrity of the swallow mechanism and may include level of arousal, ability to initiate and maintain attention during meals, tolerance for upright positioning, and/or plans for forthcoming surgical or other medical interventions.

Oral care and hygiene should be a fundamental part of every care plan at every stage of care for individuals with life-limiting conditions. Poor oral care and the presence of a feeding tube are associated with an increased risk of respiratory infection (Arnold et al., 2016; Langmore et al., 1998). Oral care increases patient comfort (NHS Ayrshire & Arran, 2017) and decreases colonization of bacteria in the oropharynx.

Value of Team Care

Care for people with life-limiting conditions and those approaching the EoL requires input from a wide range of health and social care professionals due to disease and symptom complexity, illness experience, locus of burden, and required resources. Subtle variations in any facet of an individual's situation may change the intervention and support needs dramatically. It is important to have an overall philosophy of care that keeps the patient and family at the center. This philosophy transcends any profession's scope and expertise (Sagha Zadeh et al., 2018). ASHA acknowledges that SLPs are "an integral member of the health care team and contribute significantly to the care of patients nearing end of life" (ASHA, n.d.-b).

As with supportive and palliative care services, SLPs are a consulting service, meaning the primary team (e.g., physician, nurse, social worker) makes a referral to us for guidance. One of the challenging issues for novice clinicians is that when we are called in for advice, the primary team may choose not to follow our preferred direction. Rarely is this because our input is not valued; more often, it is because the situation is complex and requires balance or trade-offs across many factors. We may find ourselves being fierce advocates for a patient where preferences go against the traditional practice in EDS intervention (Smith, 2020; Warren & Buss, 2021). For example, Warren and Buss (2021) detail a case where the SLP was positioned as both the EDS expert and the advocate for a patient wishing to eat chocolate cake near the EoL despite alleged safety risks.

SLPs routinely work in the context of interdisciplinary teams and make referrals to other professionals who can help patients. For instance, a sudden decrease in oral intake should yield a thorough dental examination, particularly for patients who cannot clearly communicate oral or dental pain. Patients with an altered diet of any sort should be referred for consultation with a dietician or nutrition service (Wright et al., 2005). The nature of a particular disease may mean that patients' nutritional needs are greater than expected—for example, with the extraneous movements of individuals with Huntington's disease (Kagel & Leopold, 1992) or the inability of the gastrointestinal system to absorb nutrients even if the oral intake appears sufficient—but the impact of declining EDS skills may further compound complications. These metabolic and systemic impairments require collaboration across professions.

Our knowledge of anatomy and physiology may contribute to spiritual care support. Even when patients are unable to swallow, they may be able to participate in religious ceremonies such as a drop of wine offered during a Seder dinner or taken in Communion (Eucharist) because the wine will be absorbed by the oral mucosa (Rourke & Leslie, 2013).

CONSIDERATIONS TOWARD THE END OF LIFE

A life-limiting condition does not mean a person is actively dying or close to death. However, in the last few days of life, there are changes in the physical system that we as health care professionals should recognize to offer appropriate support to families (Roe & George, 2016; The Gold Standards Framework, 2022). During the last week to a few days of life, it is expected that patients will show dramatic decrease in interest in eating and drinking, diminished swallow function, reduced level of arousal with fewer awake periods, and changes in respiratory patterns (see Table 1–4 in Chapter 1).

When we are called in to consult or evaluate EDS function, it is important to differentiate whether a change in EDS function is appropriate for intervention or is indicative that our goal should be to support the family with focus on patient comfort. Family members may need active support and assurance that the responsibility for care and for decision making does not lie with them alone (de Boer et al., 2015). The critical factor affecting family members' perceptions of whether their decision making surrounding a death was a good process or that they "failed" in some way largely depends on quality of communication with the health care team (Curtis & White, 2008; Handy et al., 2008).

SLPs are responsible for educating other professionals about what speech-language pathology services can offer, when it is appropriate to call us in, and when it is not. We bear responsibility for collaborating with other members of the health care team so that our dysphagia consults are appropriate based on the patient's overall health status and prognosis. Far too often, a decision to initiate tube feeding is made very late in a disease process and leads to new complications. Weissman

(2015) described this as the "Tube Feeding Death Spiral." This spiral begins with patients being admitted to the hospital for predictable brain or organ failure, due to the primary illness, and clinically they cannot sustain adequate eating, drinking, or swallowing. Following a swallowing evaluation, these patients have feeding tubes placed, which subsequently leads to increased agitation and patient removal or dislodgement of the feeding tube. The spiral continues with reinsertion of the feeding tube, successive aspiration pneumonia, and administration of intravenous antibiotics. This temporary healing in turn leads to a repeat of the agitation and feeding tube dislodgement, family conferences, and increasing distress until death (Weissman, 2015). This common pattern reinforces the necessity to recognize that the inability to maintain nutrition is usually a marker of the dying process and necessitates larger discussions with the family about overall EoL goals to limit suffering (Weissman, 2015).

There are several points at which SLPs may get involved in this sequence. For example, the onset of a new swallowing problem may yield a routine referral. Difficulties in patient care, such as administration of oral medication, may yield a referral for dysphagia assessment or a recommendation for tube feeding. When consulted, the SLP may be able to navigate alternatives to tube feeding. For example, if administration of medication is the primary concern, make a recommendation to consult with pharmacy to identify alternatives to pills such as liquid medications. The SLP should also consult with pharmacy before recommending crushing medication, which can risk dangerously altered absorption and under- or overdosing (Serrano Santos et al., 2016).

The goal of palliative and hospice care is to maximize patient comfort. In the end stages of disease, the discomfort of coughing as patients near the EoL can be substantial.

The link between oral intake and cough is not always evident to the family or the patient. Explaining that this is typical, uncomfortable, and a reason to ease the push for getting a meal down can help at this stage. Our participation as consultants in addressing EDS impairments may avert inappropriate actions or it may intrude and cause harm even if our intentions were good. We have legal and ethical duties to get it right (Brady Wagner, 2008).

SLPs have a long history of working with vulnerable patients and distressed families. Historically, SLPs have focused on rehabilitation and are used to patients improving in function over time. The same skills we use in rehabilitation to support people in difficult situations and over long periods are well suited to support those with progressive disorders and people near the EoL. We, alongside other health care professionals, can make significant contributions to patient comfort and reduce feelings of guilt or regret after the patient's death among family members (Cox, 2009). Thoughtful and timely support offered to family members faced with difficult EoL care decisions can foster acceptance and understanding of EDS functions observed in the process of dying. This support for caregivers alleviates feelings of guilt and inadequacy as they grapple with uncertainty and loss. Just as at birth, when a family needs support through a significant life change, patients and families also need support as they approach death.

ADDITIONAL RESOURCES

Increasingly, EoL and death occur behind closed doors, away from the involvement and view of friends and family. How is it, then, that clinicians can prepare themselves to work with patients and their families as they move through these critical life stages? Much of our work rests on the depth and breadth of profes-sional literature in medicine and bioethics and is accessible through most university and hospital library systems. Many palliative care and hospice resources are available online for both professionals and patients (see Appendix C for additional resources). Beyond hands-on experience and evidence-based research, there is a rich literature that represents the voices of patients, families, and health professionals. All professionals can learn from the lived experience of those who have described their journey with a life-limiting condition. Clinicians who are invited to consult with hospice or palliative care teams should collaborate closely with the lead physicians, nurses, social workers, pharmacists, and other members of the team to build knowledge and skills to support the population of patients served. Through these various forms of additional learning and exposure, clinicians can increase comfort and skill to allow for effective, empathetic care for patients and families during these crucial moments of transition.

REFERENCES

Albom, M. (2007). *Tuesdays With Morrie: An old man, a young man, and life's greatest lesson.* Little, Brown.

Ambuel, B. (2004). Responding to patient emotion #29. *Journal of Palliative Medicine, 7*(3), 473–474. https://doi.org/10.1089/10966210 41349536

Ambuel, B. (2016). *Establishing end-of-life goals: The living well interview.* Palliative Care Network of Wisconsin. https://www.mypcnow .org/fast-fact/establishing-end-of-life-goals-the-living-well-interview/

American Society of Clinical Oncology. (2019). *Long-term side effects of cancer treatment.* Cancer.net. https://www.cancer.net/survivorship/long-term-side-effects-cancer-treatment

American Speech-Language-Hearing Association. (n.d.-a). *Documentation in healthcare.* https://

www.asha.org/practice-portal/professional-issues/documentation-in-health-care/#collapse_1

American Speech-Language-Hearing Association. (n.d.-b). *End-of-life issues in speech-language pathology.* https://www.asha.org/slp/clinical/endoflife/

American Speech-Language-Hearing Association. (2016). *Scope of practice in speech-language pathology.* https://www.asha.org/policy/SP2016-00343/

Arnold, M., Liesirova, K., Broeg-Morvay, A., Meisterernst, J., Schlager, M., Mono, M. L., . . . Sarikaya, H. (2016). Dysphagia in acute stroke: Incidence, burden and impact on clinical outcome. *PLoS ONE, 11*(2), e0148424. https://doi.org/10.1371/journal.pone.0148424

Baile, W. F., Buckman, R., Lenzi, R., Glober, G., Beale, E. A., & Kudelka, A. P. (2000). SPIKES—A six-step protocol for delivering bad news: Application to the patient with cancer. *The Oncologist, 5*(4), 302–311. https://doi.org/10.1634/theoncologist.5-4-302

Banks, M., Bauer, J., Graves, N., & Ash, S. (2010). Malnutrition and pressure ulcer risk in adults in Australian healthcare facilities. *Nutrition, 26*(9), 896–901. https://doi.org/10.1016/j.nut.2009.09.024

Barbon, C., Hope, A., & Steele, C. (2017). Radiation 101: A guide for speech-language pathologists. *Perspectives of the ASHA Special Interest Groups, 2*(13), 63–72. https://doi.org/10.1044/persp2.SIG13.63

Beck, A. M., Kjaersgaard, A., Hansen, T., & Poulsen, I. (2018). Systematic review and evidence-based recommendations on texture modified foods and thickened liquids for adults (above 17 years) with oropharyngeal dysphagia—An updated clinical guideline. *Clinical Nutrition, 37*(6 Pt. A), 1980–1991. https://doi.org/10.1016/j.clnu.2017.09.002

Brady Wagner, L. C. (2008). Dysphagia: Legal and ethical issues in caring for persons at the end of life. *Dysphagia, 17*, 27–32. https://doi.org/10.1044/sasd17.1.27

Bunn, D., Jimoh, F., Wilsher, S. H., & Hooper, L. (2015). Increasing fluid intake and reducing dehydration risk in older people living in long-term care: A systematic review. *Journal American*

Medical Directors Association, 16(2), 101–113. https://doi.org/10.1016/j.jamda.2014.10.016

Carter, A. N. (2020). To what extent does clinically assisted nutrition and hydration have a role in the care of dying people? *Journal of Palliative Care, 35*(4), 209–216. https://doi.org/10.1177/0825859720907426

Chahda, L., Mathisen, B. A., & Carey, L. B. (2017). The role of speech-language pathologists in adult palliative care. *International Journal of Speech Language Pathology, 19*(1), 58–68. https://doi.org/10.1080/17549507.2016.1241301

Childers, J. (2019). *Undue influence or relational autonomy? When family members steer medical decisions.* University of Pittsburgh. https://dom.pitt.edu/wp-content/uploads/2019/10/Case-September-2019.pdf

Cox, J. (2009). Making the healing difference: Guilt and regret. *American Journal of Hospice & Palliative Medicine, 26*(1), 64–65.

Curtis, J. R., & White, D. B. (2008). Practical guidance for evidence-based ICU family conferences. *Chest, 134*(4), 835–843. https://doi.org/10.1378/chest.08-0235

Dalton, J., Rothpletz-Puglia, P., Epstein, J. B., Rawal, S., Ganzer, H., Brody, R., . . . Touger-Decker, R. (2022). Transitioning the eating experience in survivors of head and neck cancer. *Supportive Care in Cancer, 30*(2), 1451–1461. https://doi.org/10.1007/s00520-021-06526-w

de Boer, M. E., Depla, M., Wojtkowiak, J., Visser, M. C., Widdershoven, G. A. M., Francke, A. L., & Hertogh, C. M. P. M. (2015). Life-and-death decision-making in the acute phase after a severe stroke: Interviews with relatives. *Palliative Medicine, 29*(5), 451–457. https://doi.org/10.1177/0269216314563427

Dickens, C., Lambert, B. L., Cromwell, T., & Piano, M. R. (2013). Nurse overestimation of patients' health literacy. *Journal of Health Communication, 18*(Suppl. 1), 62–69. https://doi.org/10.1080/10810730.2013.825670

Dzierzanowski, T., & Mercadante, S. (2022). Constipation in cancer patients—An update of clinical evidence. *Current Treatment Options in Oncology, 23*(7), 936–950. https://doi.org/10.1007/s11864-022-00976-y

Ellis, J. (2018). Family food practices: Relationships, materiality and the everyday at the end of life. *Sociology of Health & Illness, 40*(2), 353–365. https://doi.org/10.1111/1467-9566.12606

Fan, Y., Yao, Q., Liu, Y., Jia, T., Zhang, J., & Jiang, E. (2022). Underlying causes and co-existence of malnutrition and infections: An exceedingly common death risk in cancer. *Frontiers in Nutrition, 9.* https://doi.org/10.3389/fnut.2022.814095

Flaschner, E., & Katz, D. (2015). American geriatrics society position statement on feeding tubes in advanced dementia. *Journal of the American Geriatric Society, 63*(7), 1490–1491. https://doi.org/10.1111/jgs.13554

Goldberg, L. S., & Altman, K. W. (2014). The role of gastrostomy tube placement in advanced dementia with dysphagia: A critical review. *Clinical Interventions in Aging, 9,* 1733–1739. https://doi.org/10.2147/CIA.S53153

Gozdziewski, T. H., Fabus, R. L., Geise Arroyo, C. G., Reilly Limowski, J., & Yude-Kuznetsov, J. (2019). *Goal writing for the speech-language pathologist and special educator: Bridging the gap between assessment and intervention.* Jones & Bartlett Learning.

Hallenbeck, J. (2015). *Tube feed or not tube feed?* Palliative Care Network of Wisconsin. https://www.mypcnow.org/fast-fact/tube-feed-or-not-tube-feed/

Handy, C. M., Sulmasy, D. P., Merkel, C. K., & Ury, W. A. (2008). The surrogate's experience in authorizing a do not resuscitate order. *Palliative & Supportive Care, 6*(1), 13–19. https://doi.org/10.1017/S1478951508000035

Hayes, J., & Bajzek, D. (2008). Understanding and reducing the knowledge effect: Implications for writers. *Written Communication, 25*(1), 104–118. https://doi.org/10.1177/07410883 07311209

Kagel, M. C., & Leopold, N. A. (1992). Dysphagia in Huntington's disease: A 16-year retrospective. *Dysphagia, 7*(2), 106–114. https://doi.org/10.1007/BF02493441

Kershner, M., & Askren, A. N. (2022). It's not only swallowing: A clinician primer to adult food refusal beyond dysphagia. *Current Opinion in Otolaryngology & Head & Neck Surgery,* *30*(3), 194–197. https://doi.org/10.1097/MOO.0000000000000798

Kleinman, A. (1988). *The illness narratives.* Basic Books.

Kleinman, A., Eisenberg, L., & Good, B. (1978). Culture, illness, and care: Clinical lessons from anthropologic and cross-cultural research. *Annals of Internal Medicine, 88*(2), 251–258. https://doi.org/10.7326/0003-4819-88-2-251

Kristensen, M. B., Isenring, E., & Brown, B. (2020). Nutrition and swallowing therapy strategies for patients with head and neck cancer. *Nutrition, 69,* 110548. https://doi.org/10.1016/j.nut.2019.06.028

Langmore, S. E., Terpenning, M. S., Schork, A., Chen, Y., Murray, J. T., Lopatin, D., & Loesche, W. J. (1998). Predictors of aspiration pneumonia: How important is dysphagia? *Dysphagia, 13*(2), 69–81.

Lawton, J. (2022). Counseling clients with dysphagia: A resource for clinicians. *Perspectives of the ASHA Special Interest Groups, 7*(3), 807–815. https://doi.org/10.1044/2022_PERSP-21-00263

Lawton, J., AlDuraiby, A., Terhorst, L., & Leslie, P. (2022). A survey of speech-language pathologists' use of patient medication information for patients with dysphagia. *Perspectives of the ASHA Special Interest Groups, 7*(3), 858–867. https://doi.org/10.1044/2022_PERSP-21-00268

Lazarus, C. L. (2009). Effects of chemotherapy on voice and swallowing. *Current Opinion in Otolaryngology & Head and Neck Surgery, 17*(3), 172–178. https://doi.org/10.1097/MOO.0b013e32832af12f

Lazenby-Paterson, T. (2020). Thickened liquids: Do they still have a place in the dysphagia toolkit? *Current Opinion in Otolaryngology & Head & Neck Surgery, 28*(3), 145–154. https://doi.org/10.1097/MOO.0000000000000622

Leopold, N. A., & Kagel, M. C. (1997). Dysphagia—ingestion or deglutition?: A proposed paradigm. *Dysphagia, 12*(4), 202–206. https://doi.org/10.1007/pl00009537

Leslie, P., & Broll, J. (2022). Eating, drinking, and swallowing difficulties: The impacts on, and of, religious beliefs. *Geriatrics (Basel), 7*(2), 41. https://doi.org/10.3390/geriatrics7020041

Leslie, P., Xia, B., & Yoo, J. (2021). It's not such a small world after all: The intersection of food, identity, and the speech-language pathologist. *Perspectives of the ASHA Special Interest Groups, 6*(4), 876–884. https://doi.org/10.1044/2021_PERSP-20-00276

Lippert, W. C., Chadha, R., & Sweigart, J. R. (2019). Things we do for no reason: The use of thickened liquids in treating hospitalized adult patients with dysphagia. *Journal of Hospital Medicine, 14*(5), 315–317. https://doi.org/10.12788/jhm.3141

Mannix, K. (2017). *With the end in mind: Dying, death and wisdom in an age of denial.* William Collins.

Martin, B. J. W., Corlew, M. M., Wood, H., Olson, D., Golopol, L. A., Wingo, M., & Kirmani, N. (1994). The association of swallowing dysfunction and aspiration pneumonia. *Dysphagia, 9*(1), 1–6. https://doi.org/10.1007/BF00262751

McCann, R. M., Hall, W. J., & Groth-Junker, A. (1994). Comfort care for terminally ill patients: The appropriate use of nutrition and hydration. *Journal of the American Medical Association, 272*(16), 1263–1266.

McCotter, L., Douglas, P., Laur, C., Gandy, J., Fitzpatrick, L., Rajput-Ray, M., & Ray, S. (2016). Hydration education: Developing, piloting and evaluating a hydration education package for general practitioners. *BMJ Open, 6*(12), e012004. https://doi.org/10.1136/bmjopen-2016-012004

McCurtin, A., Healy, C., Kelly, L., Murphy, F., Ryan, J., & Walsh, J. (2018). Plugging the patient evidence gap: What patients with swallowing disorders post-stroke say about thickened liquids. *International Journal of Language and Communication Disorders, 53*(1), 30–39. https://doi.org/10.1111/1460-6984.12324

Miserandino, C. (2003). *The spoon theory.* But YouDontLookSick.com. https://butyoudontlooksick.com/articles/written-by-christine/the-spoon-theory/

Morley, J. E. (2015). Dehydration, hypernatremia, and hyponatremia. *Clinics in Geriatric Medicine, 31*(3), 389–399. https://doi.org/10.1016/j.cger.2015.04.007

Nativ-Zeltzer, N., Nachalon, Y., Kaufman, M. W., Seeni, I. C., Bastea, S., Aulakh, S. S., . . . Belafsky, P. C. (2022). Predictors of aspiration pneumonia and mortality in patients with dysphagia. *Laryngoscope, 132*(6), 1172–1176. https://doi.org/10.1002/lary.29770

NHS Ayrshire and Arran. (2017). *NHS Scotland's caring for smiles: Improving the oral health of adults in care settings in line with NICE guidance and quality standards.* National Institute for Health and Care Excellence. https://www.nice.org.uk/sharedlearning/nhs-scotland-s-caring-for-smiles-improving-the-oral-health-of-adults-in-care-settings-in-line-with-nice-guidance-and-quality-standards

Oates, L. L., & Price, C. I. (2017). Clinical assessments and care interventions to promote oral hydration amongst older patients: A narrative systematic review. *BMC Nursing, 16*(4). https://doi.org/10.1186/s12912-016-0195-x

Padilla, A. H., Palmer, P. M., & Rodriguez, B. L. (2019). The relationship between culture, quality of life, and stigma in Hispanic New Mexicans with dysphagia: A preliminary investigation using quantitative and qualitative analysis. *American Journal of Speech-Language Pathology, 28*(2), 485–500. https://doi.org/10.1044/2018_ajslp-18-0061

Popkin, B. M., D'Anci, K. E., & Rosenberg, I. H. (2010). Water, hydration, and health. *Nutrition Reviews, 68*(8), 439–458. https://doi.org/10.1111/j.1753-4887.2010.00304.x

Rivelsrud, M. C., Hartelius, L., Bergstrom, L., Lovstad, M., & Speyer, R. (2022). Prevalence of oropharyngeal dysphagia in adults in different healthcare settings: A systematic review and meta-analyses. *Dysphagia.* https://doi.org/10.1007/s00455-022-10465-x

Roe, J., & George, R. (2016). When a little may be just enough? Caring for people with swallowing difficulties at the end of life, and their caregivers. *Perspectives of the ASHA Special Interest Groups, 1*(2), 89–93.

Roe, J., & Leslie, P. (2010). Beginning of the end? Ending the therapeutic relationship in palliative care. *International Journal of Speech-Language Pathology, 12*(4), 304–308. https://doi.org/10.3109/17549507.2010.485330

Rourke, N., & Leslie, P. (2013). Sacramental swallow: How swallowing informs eucharistic theology. *National Catholic Bioethics Quarterly*, *13*(2), 253–262. https://doi.org/10.5840/ncbq 201313247

Sackett, D. L., Rosenberg, W. M., Gray, J. A., Haynes, R. B., & Richardson, W. S. (1996). Evidence based medicine: What it is and what it isn't. *BMJ (Clinical research ed.)*, *312*(7023), 71–72. http://www.ncbi.nlm.nih.gov/pubmed /8555924

Sagha Zadeh, R., Eshelman, P., Setla, J., & Sadat-safavi, H. (2018). Strategies to improve quality of life at the end of life: Interdisciplinary team perspectives. *American Journal of Hospice & Palliative Care*, *35*(3), 411–416. https://doi .org/10.1177/1049909117711997

Schuetz, P., Seres, D., Lobo, D. N., Gomes, F., Kaegi-Braun, N., & Stanga, Z. (2021). Management of disease-related malnutrition for patients being treated in hospital. *Lancet*, *398*(10314), 1927–1938. https://doi.org/10 .1016/S0140-6736(21)01451-3

Serrano Santos, J. M., Poland, F., Wright, D., & Longmore, T. (2016). Medicines administration for residents with dysphagia in care homes: A small scale observational study to improve practice. *International Journal of Pharmaceutics*, *512*(2), 416–421. https://doi.org/10.1016/j .ijpharm.2016.02.036

Shune, S. E., Linville, D., & Namasivayam-MacDonald, A. (2022). Integrating family-centered care into chronic dysphagia management: A tutorial. *Perspectives of the ASHA Special Interest Groups*, *7*(3), 795–806. https://doi.org/ 10.1044/2022_PERSP-21-00314

Smith, P. (2020). Palliative care in dysphagia and dementia. *Perspectives of the ASHA Special Interest Groups*, *5*(2), 506–510. https://doi.org/ 10.1044/2020_PERSP-19-00038

Steele, S. J., Ennis, S. L., & Dobler, C. C. (2021). Treatment burden associated with the intake of thickened fluids. *Breathe (Sheff)*, *17*(1), 210003. https://doi.org/10.1183/20734735.0003-2021

Tandoh, R. (2021). *A love letter to . . . peanut butter*. Waitrose & Partners Food.

The Gold Standards Framework (2022). *Proactive identification guidance (PIG)* (7th ed.). https:// goldstandardsframework.org.uk/proactive-identification-guidance-pig

Veldee, M. S., & Peth, L. D. (1992). Can protein-calorie malnutrition cause dysphagia? *Dysphagia*, *7*(2), 86–101.

Wallin, V., Carlander, I., Sandman, P. O., Ternestedt, B. M., & Hakanson, C. (2014). Maintaining ordinariness around food: Partners' experiences of everyday life with a dying person. *Journal of Clinical Nursing*, *23*(19–20), 2748–2756. https://doi.org/10.1111/jocn.12518

Wang, C. H., Charlton, B., & Kohlwes, J. (2016). The horrible taste of nectar and honey—Inappropriate use of thickened liquids in dementia: A teachable moment. *JAMA Internal Medicine*, *176*(6), 735–736. https://doi.org/10.1001/ jamainternmed.2016.1384

Warren, A., & Buss, M. K. (2021). Death by chocolate: The palliative management of dysphagia. *Journal of Palliative Medicine, Online Ahead of Print*, pp. 1–5. https://doi.org/10.1089/jpm .2021.0487

Weissman, D. (2015). *Tube feeding and the death spiral*. Palliative Care Network of Wisconsin. https://www.mypcnow.org/fast-fact/swallow-studies-tube-feeding-and-the-death-spiral/

Wright, L., Cotter, D., Hickson, M., & Frost, G. (2005). Comparison of energy and protein intakes of older people consuming a texture modified diet with a normal hospital diet. *Journal of Human Nutrition and Diet*, *18*(3), 213–219. https://doi .org/10.1111/j.1365-277X.2005.00605.x

Wu, X. S., Miles, A., & Braakhuis, A. (2020). Nutritional intake and meal composition of patients consuming texture modified diets and thickened fluids: A systematic review and meta-analysis. *Healthcare*, *8*(4), 579–603. https://doi .org/10.3390/healthcare8040579

Xia, J. (2020). The obligation of listening: Caring for patients with chronic dysphagia through illness narratives. *Perspectives of the ASHA Special Interest Groups*, *5*(1), 231–235. https://doi .org/10.1044/2019_PERSP-19-00030

Yedidia, M. J. & MacGregor, B. (2001). Confronting the prospect of dying: Reports of terminally ill patients. *Journal of Pain and Symptom Management*, *22*(4), 807–819. https://doi.org/10.10 16/s0885-3924(01)00325-6

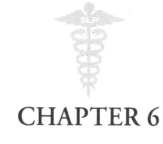

CHAPTER 6

Speech, Language, and Communication Services for Children With Life-Limiting Conditions

John Costello and Rachel Santiago

> *"Children are not small adults."* —Gillis, 2007

INTRODUCTION

Nearly 400,000 children in the United States live with severe life-limiting illnesses such as cancer, heart disease, or kidney disease and could benefit from palliative care (Center to Advance Palliative Care [CAPC], 2019). Pediatric palliative care (PPC) is not about dying; it is about helping children and families live to their fullest while facing complex medical conditions (Himelstein, 2006). To this end, speech-language pathologists (SLPs) may work with children supported by palliative care to achieve the best quality of life for patients and families. A palliative care approach encompasses physical, psychological, social, and spiritual domains of care (World Health Organization [WHO], 1990).

Historically, limited data are available to describe the role of the SLP in end-of-life (EoL) care for children. Where data are available, the literature often relates the SLP's role in dysphagia with limited information regarding communication assessment or intervention (Costello, 2009). As part of a multiphase study, Krikheli and colleagues (2020) conducted an international survey to investigate the role of SLPs working in PPC that highlighted the need for both dysphagia- and communication-focused care. Of responding SLPs, 88% identified their role in swallowing and feeding and 83% identified augmentative and alternative communication (AAC; Krikheli et al., 2020). Although SLPs receive more referrals for dysphagia when compared with referrals for communication, the frequency of consults may not accurately reflect the clinical needs of patients in palliative care (Hawksley et al., 2017).

PEDIATRIC HOSPICE AND PALLIATIVE CARE TEAMS

As described in Chapter 1, the palliative care team typically consists of multiple providers across a wide array of disciplines. PPC team members have specialty training and focus on pediatric development, medical complexities, and related resources. In addition, the PPC team may include a certified child life specialist (CLS), unique to children with life-limiting conditions. CLSs specialize in supporting children's coping, normalization, and individualized developmental needs in the context of, or response to, the physical, physiological, and emotional impact of illness and injury (Association of Child Life Professionals [ACLP], 2023). Given the importance of dynamic and interpersonal communication, CLSs and SLPs often work closely to provide interprofessional interventions.

As part of a multidisciplinary team, SLP intervention may focus on communication to (a) ensure a person's access to communication needs and preferences, (b) enhance the medical team's ability to provide adequate symptom management and engage in EoL discussions with the patient, and (c) support a family's ability to advocate for the patient's wishes and maintain social connectedness with their loved ones (Pollens, 2020). For some, communication may require AAC tools and strategies to support active decision making regarding care and quality of life. The scope of communication services for children with life-threatening illnesses is as diverse as the individuals SLPs serve.

Communication is essential, although specific needs and communication goals vary by age, medical status, life experience, and self-awareness of medical status and medical course. Engaging in conversations beyond the realities of life-limiting illness may be paramount for one child, while another is most interested in remaining emotionally connected with loved ones. For some children and their caregivers, the ability to share experiences and make meaning of their illness is of primary concern.

THE ESSENTIAL ROLE OF COMMUNICATION IN PEDIATRIC END-OF-LIFE CARE

Many considerations for adults in EoL care are relevant across ages; however, children represent a heterogeneous group with diverse needs and abilities. Given the legal age of adulthood at age 18 years in the United States, many U.S.-based practitioners defer EoL-related conversations to a child's parents or caregivers. However, it is essential to recognize that children are perceptive to the conversations around them and require the ability to think about, talk about, and comprehend developmentally appropriate and culturally aligned elements of their care, including EoL care.

When working with children who experience changes in medical status and evolving speech and language needs, SLPs must balance goals that focus on the maintenance of skills, establishing compensatory strategies, and/or providing alternative communication solutions in the context of a trajectory of decline in skills. As noted in Chapter 4, communication needs inevitably change over time from initial diagnosis through the course of disease progression. Therefore, SLPs' role to enhance communication and connections varies based on whether a referral is made early in the disease process or just days before death.

Inherent to the SLP's role in communication enhancement at EoL is creating inclusive opportunities for children to be involved in related conversations whenever appropriate. Sue and colleagues (2019) found that providers often run the risk of excluding children with complex medical and developmental needs from conversations related to death and dying. Some children may experience confusion and misinterpretation resulting from a change in routine, environment, and care. They may not adequately understand why family members are sad or why they are unable to see loved ones as frequently. Children may misinterpret their disease progression as punishment or consequence depending on their developmental understanding of illness and the dying process. Palliative care professionals recommend honest and straightforward information presented in a sensitive and devel-

opmentally appropriate way. By supporting comprehension, the SLP can promote conversations that align with family and patient goals, medical interventions, and care needs in a manner that accounts for the child's cognitive and language development and skills. For an example, see Case Study: Social Story later in this chapter. Figure 6–1 shows sample images used to support the social story.

POPULATIONS AT RISK

The etiology of a life-limiting diagnosis may be related to congenital, acquired, or progressive conditions. Given the heterogeneity of children's developmental trajectory in the

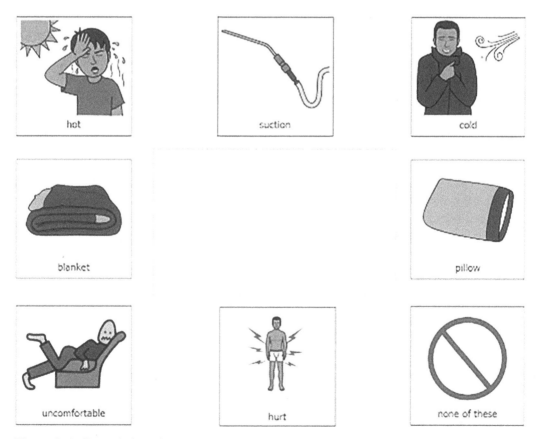

Figure 6–1. Example from Joey's communication book, which he accessed via sustained eye gaze.

context of acute or chronic illness, communication challenges may evolve throughout the child's life and particularly when the child experiences a decline in function, as occurs in EoL care. As survival rates of infants born preterm or with other complex care needs have risen with significant advances in medical care and technology over the last several decades, the prevalence of children living with complex or special care needs has increased (Cohen et al., 2011; Gilboa et al., 2016).

Congenital Disorders

Children may be born with congenital abnormalities and conditions that are functional or structural in nature. Diagnosis may occur prenatally, at the time of birth, or later in infancy or childhood. SLPs often support children with congenital anomalies to address feeding, speech and language development, and/or AAC strategies. Life expectancy associated with congenital diagnoses varies greatly and ranges from days to decades. Variability is substantial even within the same diagnostic classification. Coordinated efforts of interdisciplinary teams are typically employed early in a child's life to ensure access to needed resources, providers, and support to enhance the child's quality of life. Life-limiting congenital conditions may include:

- Genetic or inherited causes related to chromosomal differences, single gene defects, or dominant/recessively inherited conditions (e.g., mitochondrial diseases, congenital heart disease, cystic fibrosis)
- Brain abnormalities (e.g., Chiari malformation)
- Structural anatomical defects during fetal development, including congenital heart conditions, organ dysplasia, neural tube defects (e.g., spina bifida), and other

structural anomalies of the brain and spinal cord
- Environmental causes, including deficits related to adverse medication, substance, or chemical exposure in utero
- Prematurity, pregnancy, and/or perinatal complications

Acquired Conditions

Conditions such as respiratory infections, spinal cord injury, brain injury due to anoxic episodes, accidental ingestions, stroke, neuroimmune demyelinating disorders, cancers, and other diseases may become life-limiting conditions and each may render a child's communication vulnerable.

Progressive Disorders

Conditions without curative treatment may be or become progressive, resulting in neurodegeneration in cognitive and/or motor domains over time. In some children with progressive diagnoses such as Batten's disease, muscular dystrophy, or mucopolysaccharidosis, communication deficits may begin early in life, prompting referral for SLP services and implementation of tailored strategies to address functional speech, language, and communication skills. Motor neuron diseases in children are progressive neurological disorders affecting muscle activity including breathing, moving, speaking, and swallowing. Cognition in children with motor neuron diseases may remain intact throughout the life span (e.g., Duchenne muscular dystrophy, spinal muscular atrophy, Friedreich's ataxia). Some neurodegenerative diseases affect multiple body structures and systems including cognition (e.g., Leigh's disease, juvenile Huntington's disease, chronic HIV, MELAS or mitochondrial encephalomyopathy, lactic acidosis, stroke-like episodes, Niemann-Pick disease, cerebral adrenoleukodystrophy; Chiu et al., 2022).

BARRIERS AND CONSIDERATIONS TO SUPPORT COMMUNICATION FOR CHILDREN NEARING THE END OF LIFE

Children of all ages and skills can be keen observers with innate curiosities and perspectives about the world around them. A child's mood can be directly reflected from their parents or caregivers, prompting grown-ups to shield their children from difficult or scary information. Interactions with children in an EoL context often stem from a dynamic interplay among their unique and individual developmental profile, needs, wishes, and priorities together with those of their caregivers and providers.

When a child experiences a changing body and mind that directly impacts their ability to participate in meaningful interactions, SLPs can support the delivery of information in a developmentally appropriate manner. The SLP may also bolster the child's capacity for expression to reflect their inner thoughts and states of being in a way that is thoughtfully aligned with their development and with the goals and priorities of the child and their family. SLPs should consider the range of spiritual, emotional, psychological, physical, and developmental needs of each child to support meaningful interactions.

How Children Understand Pain, Illness, and Death

"Children are not small adults" is a highly regarded phrase in pediatric medicine (Gil-lis & Loughlan, 2007). There is perhaps no instance greater to apply this wisdom than when working with a child with a life-limiting disease. For the SLP, this perspective is consistent with the importance of the phrase "the work of childhood is play" (Piaget, 1951). These expressions highlight that SLPs must provide developmentally and culturally appropriate intervention for children living with a life-limiting illness. To do so, the SLP must appreciate children's developmental understanding of pain, death, and dying. How a child describes, localizes, and copes with their pain and illness will vary; thus, the SLP's role is to support appropriate information delivery that is consistent with the child's comprehension and to provide tools for expression that allow the child to communicate their pain and other messages related to their unique circumstance, capacity, and needs.

> "Understanding illness is primarily determined by cognitive maturation. Logical concepts such as the cause of illness, the necessity of treatment, and the role of medical personnel are often beyond the inherent developmental ability of the young patient. Comprehension of these issues will become more complex and realistic as the patient's cognitive processes mature. Therefore, understanding is an evolving process, and educational material must fit each child's level."
>
> —Brewster, 1982

Death and mortality are understood differently across developmental stages (Himebauch, et al., 2008). Therefore, SLPs must consider a child's developmental perspective in ongoing assessment and intervention to inform goals and interpret a child's response to information. If alternative communication tools and strategies are needed, appropriate vocabulary selection and symbolic representations must be available to support the child's ability to ask questions, comment, and participate in care.

For this discussion, we will reference *developmental* age instead of chronological age, as our clinical experience reveals that many children we have worked with are developmentally younger than their chronological age. It is essential that therapists are cognizant of each child's developmental understanding of pain, illness, and death.

There is no understanding of the concept of death for a child developmentally younger than 2 years of age (Himebauch, et al., 2008). Babies and children under 2 recognize and respond to distress, changes in the environment, unpredictable schedules, and lack of routine. The SLP may support a child and family to create consistent and predictable routines. Visual supports and social stories using photos or symbols to support comprehension and discussion about daily tasks and activities supplement consistency and routine. Developmentally young children may be supported with tools that allow them to call for attention and solicit a loved one through simple voice output technology and single switches.

Developmental Age 2 to 5 Years Old

Children who are developmentally 2 to 5 years of age do not understand abstract concepts such as "forever" and do not grasp that death is permanent and irreversible (Himebauch, et al., 2008). While the child can communicate discomfort and pain, they cannot always identify the source or location. Children at this age want to talk about the "whys" of the world and need to be supported to ask questions about their experiences and illness. Having a sense of control is vital for children at this age.

Developmental Age 5 to 7 Years Old

At the developmental age of 5 to 7, a child still does not understand the reason for pain or illness, but instead demonstrates "magical thinking" characterized by believing death and illness can be caused by thoughts or actions. Children may blame themselves or their behavior for illness (Himebauch, et al., 2008), associate illness as a form of punishment (Eiser, 1985), or believe their parents and loved ones can "fix" their illness. An example many have witnessed is a child crying inconsolably on the playground after falling and skinning a knee and soliciting a parent to "kiss the boo-boo," resulting in a quick recovery and return to play. For the critically ill child who experiences magical thinking and has limited communication skills, it is critical that they gain the ability to request attention from loved ones and be able to ask for comfort or reassurance. The SLP must ensure a child has the vocabulary and facility to express fear, communicate anxiety, solicit parents and loved ones for comfort, and seek explanation and protection. Figure 6–2 provides an example of images that convey these requests.

In a study focused on identifying appropriate vocabulary for discussing pain, Johnson and colleagues (2016) interviewed typically developing children ages 6 to 9 to develop a list of core and fringe vocabulary related to pain concepts. They described multiple types of vocabulary functions, which are essential considerations in supporting such discussions, including words to (a) describe pain, (b) direct others' actions, (c) describe pain location, (d) describe causes of pain, (e) describe strategies used to cope with pain, (f) reflect on strategies of how the pain could have been prevented, and (g) indicate the consequences of pain or injury and its influence on activities and participation.

Though pain-related vocabulary lists have been validated, working with patients and families is imperative to identify personally relevant vocabulary and messages. In addition, each child's illness, tolerance, interventions, and coping skills will vary, and require nuanced support for participation in pain-related discussions.

Developmental Age 7 to 12 Years Old

In the 7- to 12-year-old developmental range, children understand that death is final, irreversible, and universal. A child in this developmental range can typically localize their pain, understand that germs cause illness, and believe staff's response depends on how well they express pain. With this same reasoning, some children may withhold the expression of pain to avoid interventions (Brewster, 1982).

By age 7, children may associate pain outcomes with concrete solutions such as medicine, bandages, ointments, or other tangible interventions. They may also begin to use a pain rating scale functionally. An example of a developmentally appropriate scale is the Wong-Baker FACES Pain Rating Scale (Wong-Baker FACES Foundation, n.d.). Children at this age can communicate comfort and pain, location, intensity, and differentiate type of discomfort (e.g., nausea versus ache versus itchy). It is important for children in this developmental range to exert control and be able to communicate their symptoms and needs, ask questions, and collaborate in their care. Figure 6–3 shows some examples of pictures that allow a child to show where it hurts and what they perceive their needs to be.

Developmental Age 13 Years and Older

Children who are 13 years and older developmentally understand there are multiple causes of illness. At this developmental age, adolescents understand that the body may respond to many different factors, the causes of illness, and that caregivers act to support them with necessary intent and empathy. At this more

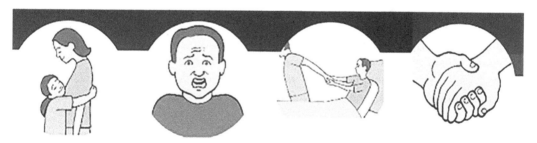

Figure 6–2. Example AAC board for expressing fear, communicating anxiety, and asking for comfort and reassurance.

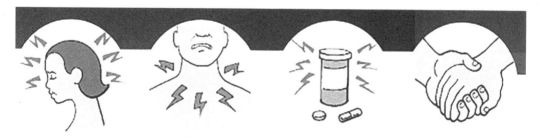

Figure 6–3. Example AAC board for communicating pain, location, and need for comfort.

mature stage, a child may be eager to ask questions, interact with staff, and understand the intent of intervention. At this level of interest and engagement, it is necessary to ensure the adolescent has the tools to communicate their questions and ideas. Typical messages of importance may include:

- How am I doing?
- Will I be okay?
- What is the plan?
- What is that medicine for?
- Will this hurt or make me nauseous?
- How long will I need to take this medication?
- How are you doing?
- When will the tube come out?
- Can I eat anything today?

At this developmental stage it is crucial that the child develops health literacy through access to relevant vocabulary in communication tools and is included in discussions and decision making as is developmentally appropriate. Many children living with complex medical conditions, who have experienced frequent hospitalizations and lengthy stays, become intimately familiar with medical parlance and engage with apparent sophistication in topics related to illness, treatment, recovery, and even death. At times the apparent command of "hospital vocabulary" can mask deficits in comprehension. Closely scrutinizing a child's authentic comprehension of their medical status is critical. Opportunities to review medical information and allow for questions are essential (see Figure 6–4, for example).

Chloe, a 5.5-year-old child with advanced pontine glioma, had experienced multiple hospitalizations and aggressive treatment regimes. When treatments were determined to be ineffective and her cancer fatal, Chloe's parents requested complete transparency and open discussion regarding death. Chloe's observed responsiveness to this was mature and interactive, and she increasingly initiated a conversation about her death and discussed her current and anticipated losses in neurological function, medications, and medical management tools and how unavoidable changes in the tumor would lead to death. Despite her apparent maturity and comprehension of her disease and fate, Chloe, who could not independently walk, observed a child driving a power wheelchair through the

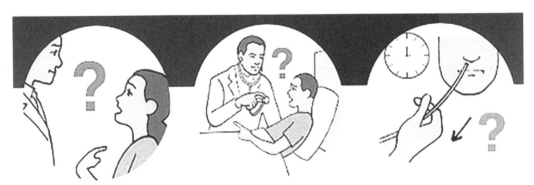

Figure 6–4. Example AAC board for assessing a child's comprehension of medical status and need for medical information.

corridor. She drew her father's attention to the power chair and asked, "After I die, will you get me one of those chairs so I can go to school?"

The father reported to the medical staff that it was at that moment he realized his daughter's understanding of death was more like the movie *The Matrix*, where there are parallel universes, as opposed to an authentic and mature understanding of her death.

Psychosocial Needs of the Dying Child

The psychosocial needs of a child who has a life-limiting condition are complex (University of California San Diego, 2020). Previously identified needs (UCSD, 2020) are expanded and considered in the context of speech-language pathology services and summarized in Table 6–1.

Time to Be a Child

As previously referenced, the work of childhood is play. Within their ability, children need to engage in age-appropriate activities, such as watching television, reading, playing games, or exploring the outdoors. Infants through young adults appreciate the ability to access play however possible through the EoL. Caregivers also often prioritize play experiences to preserve joy and normalcy for children despite physiological symptoms a child may experience during their illness. "Children need support, entertainment, and jokes and do not want to be treated like a sick child," according to nurses interviewed for a study focused on the needs of children with terminal illnesses (Adistie et al., 2020).

Children nearing EoL may experience fluctuating mental status, physical skills, and communication abilities, and require that the SLP work collaboratively with family and other professionals, such as physical therapists,

Five-year-old Pietro enjoyed playing games with the staff early in his hospitalization with astrocytoma, such as hiding under his bedsheets or pretending he was asleep when staff entered the room and then calling out "boo" to scare them. The hospital staff, ranging from nurses and doctors to environmental service workers, would respond by feigning concern for his whereabouts or being frightened by his outburst of "boo." As symptoms progressed to loss of functional speech and reduced gross and fine motor movements, Pietro's hospital room was engineered to support independent play. A simple voice output communication aid was pro-grammed with the verbal message "Boo" or "You can't find me" to be activated with a gross movement of his right wrist after his parents covered him with the bedsheets. Similarly, a single-switch modified battery-operated water cannon allowed Pietro to activate water flow when a staff member entered the room. His delight was evident through smile and raised eyebrows even at an advanced stage of disease progression. Pietro's response to humor and play with the water cannon caused hospital staff to support ongoing water play, and they positioned a mop and paper towels inside his bedspace for use as needed.

Table 6–1. Psychosocial Needs of Children With Life-Limiting Conditions and the Role of Speech-Language Pathology Intervention

Theme	Role of the Speech-Language Pathologist
Time to be a child	Engage child in age-appropriate activities whenever possible
Control and autonomy	Avoid a sense of powerlessness. It is essential for children to remain engaged and less fearful in care.
Talking about illness	Provide vocabulary suitable for the child's care needs, self-expression, and direction of care. Truthful expression aids comprehension and minimizes confusion, isolation, and loneliness.
Communication of fear and anger	Recognize behavior as communication and support healthy expression of feelings and emotions
Expression of depression and withdrawal	Support strategies to cope and gain comfort
Wish fulfillment	Provide hope and joy through the expression of wishes and positive memories
Spiritual/cultural preferences	Ensure access to and appropriate means to participate in spiritual and cultural practices
Collaboration in communication options	Engage child and family in selection of communication tools and strategies for current and future use. Learning options and guiding others with what feels most comfortable may support the most effective medical care and social connectedness.
Message banking	Record the child's speech and voice to allow authentic representation of self and support participation and engagement
Technoconnectedness	Maintain social connectedness and reduce isolation
Normalization	Preserve routines and tasks to support coping and engagement
Not alone in dying/ maintaining social connectedness	Support continued social connectedness and maintain special social closeness through disease progression
Reflection on positive life events	Encourage family to share and recount enjoyable life experiences through stories and photos. Reminiscing allows child and family to engage beyond illness and loss.
Expression of legacy	Create memories and mementos for the child to give to others, contributes to child's knowledge that others will remember them
Creating social stories	Support comprehension and provide a meta-view of relationships, illness, and legacy

Note. Themes are drawn from review of the literature (Adistie et al., 2020; UCSD, 2020) and the authors' clinical experiences.

occupational therapists, and CLSs, to meet the child's changing needs and support alternative access to play, routines, and activities. Continued access to play as a positive experience is paramount rather than children abandoning their efforts to participate in a once-joyous activity. Communication boards should depict options for play, directives, and related comments that may enhance child-directed engagement during their preferred play activities.

Control and Autonomy

As children near EoL, they may require care across varied settings. Each setting offers varied independence, control, and autonomy. In the home setting, children have increased access to familiar partners, personal belongings, and inclusion in different contexts, such as attending religious services, participating in peer interactions, and going to parks. On the other hand, children who require a higher level of care may have more restrictions in a home environment or experience frequent inpatient admissions.

Children in the health care setting are often subject to psychological trauma because they lack control of their environment; this trauma may surface as anxiety, aggression, anger, or other expressions of emotion (Lerwick, 2016). The sense of helplessness, coupled with fear and pain, can cause children to feel powerless in health care and other settings. Trauma and strong emotional responses can delay necessary medical treatment, require longer interventions, and reduce patient satisfaction (Brinkman-Stoppelenburg, 2014).

In the medical setting, children may be disoriented as they experience a loss of control and autonomy as familiar and unfamiliar caregivers take over their bodies. Bereaved parents reported patient inclusion and a strong relationship between the family members and health care providers as high priorities as children's health declined (Snaman et al., 2016). Parents, family members, and other personal caregivers highly value professionals who spent time without being rushed, listened empathetically, and created a therapeutic alliance.

Children find safety and can understand the world around them better when they can exert a level of control that is (at least sometimes) honored by the adults in their life. While children have little control while

As 10-year-old Ellie's medical condition deteriorated and family financial circumstances required that both parents continue to work, Ellie demonstrated increased anger when her parents left her bedside. While they tried to stagger their work shifts so someone was always at the bedside, this did not always work. Ellie began to resist falling asleep. She expressed anger with her care team when told that sleep would make her feel better. Ellie resisted medications when her parents were absent and would state "no sleep" through teary eyes. When one or both parents were present and committed to sleeping at the bedside, Ellie would readily sleep, most often holding her parent's hand. Ellie did not articulate the source of her fear verbally, but when using a simple communication board, she pointed to "afraid" + "sleep" + "die" + "Mom and Dad" + "go away." She confirmed that she feared dying alone, specifically without her parents present. In light of Ellie's rapidly failing status, her parents made the tough decision to take leave without pay from work for the remaining 27 days of her life.

they are in the hospital, SLPs can engineer opportunities to restore control. For example, communication tools that allow a child to direct the behavior of others; choose and modify schedules; tell people to "go away," "leave me alone," or "come back in 15 minutes"; choose from items on a dinner menu; or select the television station can provide control and agency to a child who otherwise feels helpless.

Talking About Illness

Many terminally ill children might vacillate between wanting to know details about their illness and not wanting to acknowledge they are sick (Wolfelt, 2022). As a result, children may feel alone, isolated, or confused without an opportunity to talk about their prognosis. The American Academy of Pediatrics (2016) outlines the importance of truthful expression of care by providers at every stage of intervention and development. In young children, this may include being honest about the medical items in the room or the effects of medication (e.g., "You have some tubes in your body right now. This tube helps give your belly food and water. This tube helps you to breathe so your body does not have to work too hard"). Children who benefit from visuals to support comprehension might understand anticipated medical interventions, symptoms, and procedures through pictures, demonstration, play, or stories.

Older children may be able to understand more direct and sophisticated medical terminology and/or information, with or without supplemental visuals. They may also be able to ask more specific questions about *why* a specific medication is being delivered, *how* a specific treatment will help them, or even *when* they may die. Many children with life-limiting conditions may have extremely high health literacy and exposure to medical terminology, concepts, and contexts. Some children with reduced speech output may have robust knowledge about their condition and care needs, while another child with age-appropriate speech-language skills may have limited experience in health care settings or symptoms, procedures, and vocabulary related to their diagnosis. The SLP is tasked with assessing the child's speech-language skills and the health literacy of their pediatric patients to ensure appropriate access to expressive/receptive communication tools and strategies that serve their needs and meet them where they can engage.

> Before losing the ability to speak consistently, Rachel's mother expressed distress that Rachel asked her regularly, "Am I still dying? "She highlighted that Rachel did not seem distressed by the answer still being "yes" and appeared to carry on with her play after being answered. When Rachel's speech and motor skills became extremely compromised, a simple voice output aid was used at her mother's request, programmed with the message "Am I still dying?" recorded by Rachel's cousin. Her mother indicated that, while it is highly distressing to answer the question, she realized that it somehow helped Rachel cope with what would otherwise be an unknown scenario.

Lyman and colleagues (2008) note that dying children express concern about what will happen to family pets and their belongings once they are gone. Opportunities to discuss these concerns and assurance that a plan is in place may comfort a child and help them to cope with their illness.

Six-year-old Anna self-initiated a written list of jobs for her siblings, assigning jobs such as feeding the dog, cleaning the toy room, and getting the mail from the front hall basket. A Velcro board was created with photos of her siblings and parents and symbols for each job. Daily, Anna assigned and reassigned jobs. Notably, when her father would tell her that he did not want the job of walking the dog, she would immediately assign it to him while half smiling and looking at her father.

Communication of Fear or Anger

Children may express anger related to the change in their routine, the inability to participate in previously enjoyable activities, restrictions on social engagement, and the loss of skill and function. These responses can be compounded by fear of dying, especially of dying alone. Often, children are reassured, comforted, and cope better with complex information when allowed to identify and express their true feelings. By providing opportunities for such expression, the SLP can open avenues for gaining needed comfort and compassion, and support more nuanced coping.

Expression of Depression and Withdrawal

Loss of control, loss of prior function, and changes in routines, coupled with a reduced ability to communicate these concerns, may result in withdrawal and feelings of anxiety and depression. Children continually develop coping skills and integrate individual experiences, learned behaviors, and information from others to navigate difficult circumstances. Given that children do not always express emotions in the same way as adults, fear and anxiety may be expressed through anger, combativeness, physical communication, or withdrawal (Brewer, 2020). The SLP must be cognizant of this and, whenever possible, provide vocabulary that allows the child to identify their emotions and initiate conversation. The SLP should collaborate with other members of the team including CLSs, developmental psychologist, social workers, or other mental health specialist members of the team.

Wish Fulfillment

Adolescents and young adults may prioritize the expression of wishes to loved ones (Sansom-Daly et al., 2020). The literature highlights the need to enable and empower adolescents and recognize their role in self-determination and decision making (Snaman et al., 2016). Supporting older children and adolescents to communicate their wishes and to collaborate with the medical team to fulfill a wish is a powerful way to provide hope and joy for the child and create positive memories for the family.

Throughout the last year of her illness, 19-year-old Sandra had stated her desire to have a rose tattoo on her shoulder. As her ability to speak became compromised, Sandra proactively worked with the SLP to create a communication board with symbols and text. One of her first chosen messages was, "I want a tattoo." In her last weeks of life, Sandra used her communication board to request a tattoo repeatedly. Finally, to honor her wish, Sandra's family and the medical team arranged for Sandra to meet with a tattoo artist, who designed and applied a rose tattoo on her shoulder.

Spiritual and Cultural Preferences

Maintaining spiritual and cultural preferences and practices is essential to communication in pediatrics and EoL care. For many families, religiosity, prayer, and spirituality are integral to family systems and conversations before, during, and after the child's death. However, supporting these conversations for children often depends on the child's and family's specific practices, beliefs, and preferences. For example, children may wish to participate in prayers in an accessible manner. For children unable to produce speech at EoL, this may be achieved through the activation of voice-output communication aids or a speech-generating device with recorded whole prayers or responses (e.g., "Amen" following recitation). For others, the ability to request prayer recited by others or participate in meditative experiences may be essential to their quality of life.

The SLP may also help to uphold a child's and family's specific implementations of cultural practices, rituals, and beliefs. This may include learning how family members communicate with one another, participating in and communicating about familial rituals and bonding experiences, and integrating topics such as traditional foods, cultural perspectives, and community events. SLPs may collaborate with community spiritual leaders and/or hospital chaplains to support individual patients and their families. SLPs should practice compassionate curiosity to understand the child's and family's spiritual preferences and identify ways to incorporate these beliefs and practices into communication strategies.

Anticipatory Grief

Anticipatory grief occurs before death. Parents and loved ones of a child with a life-limiting illness may grieve the loss of current meaningful activities, changes in interactions, and/or future losses or what could have been. The SLP may be instrumental in guiding the child and family to create authentic and meaningful interactions that the surviving loved ones may remember, review, and cherish. At the same time, engaging activities may bring joy and relief to the child, who may be concerned for those left behind (Lyman, 2008). Even if a child cannot fully participate in activities as they were once able to, supporting participation in the best way possible may be of value. For nonspeaking or minimally speaking children, the SLP may be instrumental in supporting the child's participation and creating an outcome that will be meaningful to the grieving family member in the present and in the future.

As Amy continued to lose skills, her father would play games with her by pretending he did not know how to do something and asking Amy to help him by explaining it. For example, one of Amy's jobs had been to feed the family dog. One of the questions she had asked her father was "Who is going to feed Pepper (the dog)?" He would say, "I will" and feign forgetting something or getting information wrong. For example, he would say "Oh, Pepper eats lettuce, right?" and Amy would exclaim "Nooo, you have to give him dry dog food and mix in water and cheese bits!" Working with the SLP, Amy created a board with visual directions for her father to follow. She instructed her father to take photos of several items, such as the cabinet where the dog food is kept, the bag of dog food, and the string cheese in the refrigerator. The SLP used the photos to create a communication board with the photos in sequence to complete the task using Amy's instructions.

COMMUNICATION EVALUATION FOR CHILDREN WITH TERMINAL ILLNESS

Palliative care presents a paradigm shift for clinicians accustomed to care focused on rehabilitation or habilitation (Krikheli et al., 2021). While the knowledge and skills of the SLP are essential, the process of assessment and intervention with a palliative care focus for children differs from more traditional SLP assessment and intervention methods. Multiple domains of speech, language, voice, and social communication must be assessed and reassessed in the context of medical status and the child's developmental stage. Several domains of communication can be evaluated simultaneously in one or more sessions. While working with children with life-limiting conditions and their families, a softer and more nuanced approach to speech-language evaluation is recommended. Evaluation should prioritize warmth, compassion, and sensitivity over completed checklists and comprehensive, detailed assessment and data collection. As previously highlighted, it is ideal for the SLP to be involved as early as possible, especially if future communication challenges are anticipated. Dynamic assessment is prioritized through reevaluating skills and by responsiveness to intervention, needs, wishes, and goals over time. Children and their families are collaborators in the process and can be empowered and given hope through active engagement and identification of potentially supportive strategies that promote participation in medical and nonmedical discussions, enhance expressive and receptive communication, and promote social connection.

Context

Depending on the child's condition and timing of diagnosis, SLPs may evaluate a child's communication needs at varied points in their life and illness trajectory. Children with baseline communication impairments may already be working with an SLP. If already receiving services, SLPs may work with their clients in an outpatient setting such as early intervention, private practice, outpatient hospital clinic, or school. If the SLP already has a relationship with the child and family, existing goals can be adapted or supplemented to support the maintenance skills or to accommodate changes in skills over time. In other instances, children may receive the initial diagnosis of a life-limiting condition while hospitalized. For new-onset conditions, the child and family may first encounter speech-language services in the acute care hospital setting such as an emergency department, intensive care unit, or inpatient hospital unit.

Some children may require SLP services for months or years as an outpatient or may receive SLP support for a short duration during an inpatient stay. Some children may remain in inpatient care from the time of diagnosis through the EoL. Typically, children nearing the EoL are not admitted to inpatient rehabilitation settings; however, in some cases, SLPs in such contexts may receive referrals for assessment or intervention depending on staffing and goals of inpatient rehabilitation services or related to administrative connection to a broader pediatric medical care facility.

SLPs may encounter patients who fluctuate between inpatient, home, and community environments and who may receive services in more than one of these settings. Some families may enroll in a hospice program that employs or contracts with SLPs to provide EoL care and support for communication and/or dysphagia. Hospice-specific services can occur in the child's home, a hospital setting, or a hospice facility.

Direct and Indirect Assessments

Dynamic assessment is completed in short and frequent visits tailored to meet the child's alertness, comfort, energy, and priority related to other care needs. Formal and standardized testing are rarely, if ever, employed. Instead, reports from primary nursing staff, medical record review, ongoing parental and/or primary care provider reports, and observation of the child's engagement, alertness/arousal, changes in attention and participation, respiration rate, and current use of aided and unaided communication strategies are all measures used to determine appropriate communication interventions (Costello et al., 2010).

A dynamic feature-matching process, which focuses on matching the most effective communication tools and strategies to a child's strengths, needs, and skills is used (Shane & Costello, 1996) and must be revisited at each stage of disease progression to establish and maintain opportunities for communication success. Essential elements of an evaluation for children with life-limiting conditions nearing EoL include:

- Building rapport
- Information gathering (i.e., through the interview, conversation, and child-directed play and interactions)
- Observation and informal assessment procedures
- Formal procedures, if indicated: These may include an oral mechanism examination, collecting a language sample, and evaluation subtests if appropriate (for example, aphasia subtests in the event of a stroke or other neurological changes)
- Feature matching for communication support across domains of assessment (Table 6–2)
- Trial of supportive strategies, including AAC

Assessment outcomes rely on the SLP, patient, and family achieving a shared understanding of current status and goals and thus requires discussion about prognosis. Common reasons practitioners may avoid open discussions with patients and caregivers about EoL care can include prognostic uncertainty, difficulty ascertaining the patient's and family's readiness to participate, and fear of causing undue distress. A leading cause of avoidance by SLPs may be feeling unprepared for difficult conversations, which can lead to missed opportunities to provide important and appropriate patient support during a delicate and valued time. The palliative care literature offers recommendations to support clinicians when approaching the topic of EoL. These recommendations are detailed in the following sections and include (a) establishing patient and family goals, (b) leading with compassionate curiosity, and (c) calibrating your communication style (see also Chapter 1).

Establish Patient and Family Goals

Gathering information from the family, patient, and multidisciplinary team members about the child's current skills and presentation is an essential initial step in assessment. Identifying what is working and what is challenging through collaborative discussions can help guide goal-oriented discussions. For children nearing EoL, it is crucial for the SLP to guide conversations related to patient and family goals with sensitivity and care. Goals may be related to skills (e.g., speech, language, and cognitive skills) or quality of life (e.g., maintaining social connections, continuing to participate in schooling, spending as much time at home as possible, reducing pain and suffering). In addition, the SLP should support patients and families to maintain skills as indicated, identify compensatory strategies, implement communication repair strategies, recommend and implement AAC strategies, and enhance communication and interactions across settings and partners through supportive partner training.

Table 6–2. Domains of Assessment With Feature-Matching Considerations for Augmentative and Alternative Communication Strategies in End-of-Life Care for Children

Assessment Domain	Assessment Considerations	Feature Matching Considerations and Options for System Selection
Cognition: alertness, awareness, orientation, premorbid status	• Nursing staff report • Ability to remain awake • Ability to follow commands • Memory encoding, recall, and retention • Attention • Problem solving • Delirium	• Frequency, timing, complexity of assessment, instruction, and strategies introduced • Use of memory book and/or orientation strategies • Train partner in strategies for communication (e.g., redirection, ways to promote attention, visual schedules) • Implement delirium prevention and management strategies
Sensory systems	General Sensory Considerations • Sensitivities to touch, light, sound, taste, smell Vision • Premorbid vision • Current vision • Availability of visual aids Hearing • Premorbid hearing • Current hearing Accessibility of Sensory Adaptations • Availability and access to adaptive equipment such as corrective lenses, hearing aids, FM systems • Individual's ability to don and doff adaptive equipment such as glasses or hearing aids independently	• Determine how to represent language concepts through visual channel (e.g., line drawings, photographs, symbols, text) • Explore visual accommodations (e.g., high-contrast displays of pictures and/or text, use of backlighting) • Assess sensory capacity for use of aided communication strategies (e.g., communication boards, speech-generating devices) • Explore augmented input (e.g., live transcription) • Explore environmental accommodations to support visual access, hearing, and listening • Facilitate use of hearing aids, FM system, or other assisted listening device • Consider partner-assisted auditory scanning • Use patient-to-partner typing system
Language comprehension, production, literacy screening	Language comprehension	• Determine the approximate level of comprehension, vocabulary needs, and how to represent vocabulary • Consider augmented input (e.g., speech to text, writing/typing to the patient, picture-communication boards to signal the topic of conversation)

continues

Table 6–2. *continued*

Assessment Domain	Assessment Considerations	Feature Matching Considerations and Options for System Selection
Language comprehension, production, literacy screening *continued*	Non-English speaker	• Structure communication tools in primary language with English alongside to support staff understanding • Use picture-based communication tools • Digital voice recording to translate basic care needs and other often-used messages
	Ability to answer yes/no questions	Establish a reliable yes/no/maybe system or strategy
	Literacy screening	• Written words • Alphabet for novel messages • Picture-based system • Comprehensive speech-generating device that supports spelling • Typing efficiency strategies
Motor access: assess in different positions	Gestures/pantomime	• Natural gestures • Gestural codes • Yes/no signals
	Control/Access • Ability to directly select a target (e.g., via pointing, keyboard use, whole-hand approximation, eye gaze, use of pointers)	• Signal for yes/no • Standard or adapted nurse call system • Consider use of a single message system for attention/assistance • Size and layout of word/picture board • Interface for electronic devices (e.g., keyboard, key guard, dynamic display, eye gaze) • Nonelectronic eye gaze strategy
	Ability to use indirect selection strategies	• Technology-based scanning • Partner-assisted scanning
	Ability to write/draw	• Alphabet or whole-word communication board • Pen and paper • Whiteboard and marker • Writing tablets
Speech production	Vocal function and loudness	• Amplification (e.g., wearable voice amplifier) • Electrolarynx • Consider use of a single message system for attention/assistance

Table 6–2. *continued*

Assessment Domain	Assessment Considerations	Feature Matching Considerations and Options for System Selection
Speech production *continued*	Moderately compromised intelligibility	• Letter cueing/topic cueing • Writing/typing • Word- or symbol-based communication board • Communication repair strategies • Speech-generating device • Voice and message banking
	Nonspeaking or severely compromised intelligibility	• Alphabet board • Word/symbol communication board • Speech-generating device • Consider the use of a single message system for attention/assistance
Vocabulary selection	• Patient needs • Patient personality • Patient interests • Medical, personal, and psychosocial needs	• Premade commercial boards • Custom boards • Communication book • Spelling with an alphabet board • Speech-generating device (simple to complex)
Environmental assessment	• Lighting • Noise • Physical environment	• Ensure adequate lighting to see the communication board • Verify voice output from communication devices is audible above background noise • Mount or position communication tools in space available, wheelchair, or other positioning factors to accommodate easy access by the child, family, and staff
Communication partners	• Native language • Hearing status • Literacy level • Caregiver burden	Design to support communication success with nonliterate, deaf or hard of hearing, or non-English-speaking family members.
Prognosis	Potential for progressive loss of speech, motor, sensory, cognition, and/or language skills	Introduce tools and strategies that meet current needs and can adapt with child and family as needs change. Example: introducing a partner-assisted scanning strategy to support familiarity, even if not immediately needed

continues

Table 6–2. *continued*

Assessment Domain	Assessment Considerations	Feature Matching Considerations and Options for System Selection
Documentation and staff training	• Team member responsibilities and availability • The ability for others to carry over recommendations • Dissemination of information	• Consider the diversity of the team and time demands • Ensure caregivers and providers are educated on the setup and/or implementation of aided communication strategies • Support carryover • Support maintenance and troubleshooting of equipment

Source: Adapted from Costello, J. M., Patak, L., & Pritchard, J. (2010). Communication vulnerable patients in the pediatric ICU: Enhancing care through augmentative and alternative communication. *Journal of Pediatric Rehabilitation Medicine, 3*(4), 289–301. https://doi.org/10.3233/PRM-2010-0140

Over time, the SLP may also support the adaptation and modification of goals, strategies, and participation based on the child's evolving needs and disease progression.

Some children, especially young adults, are interested in and able to participate in care plans, medical decisions, and establishing advance directives. The SLP should uphold and integrate personal identity, cultural values, spiritual beliefs, and neurodiverse considerations into intervention and continuously support access to developmentally appropriate language and messages about goals of care and plans of care. In consultation with the palliative care team and/or CLSs, several resources are available to support children, adolescents, young adults, and families in these conversations (Five Wishes, 2023). "My Wishes" is an

---

When Sam's clinical status changed, she endorsed a desire to participate in discharge planning to home hospice. Sam, who had cerebral palsy and dysarthric speech at baseline, had undergone tracheostomy placement several months prior to a cardiac arrest, precluding her from using speech due to ventilator settings. While in the hospital, along with her family members and clinical staff, a bedside feature-matched assessment was conducted. Shortly after the assessment, Sam began to use partner-assisted spelling and a customized communication book to communicate. Though only 16 years old, Sam had always participated actively in her school and community. When the palliative care team discussed advance care planning, she indicated her desire to be actively included in these discussions. The SLP, CLS, and palliative care team joined Sam and her mom at the bedside. The SLP supported partner-assisted scanning with Sam's custom letter board. Through spelling, Sam asked questions about her prognosis, engaged in meaningful conversations about risks and benefits of proposed medical interventions, and ultimately expressed clear wishes about her care, location of care, and specific advance directives.

advance care planning document designed to support school-aged children and "Voicing My Choices" is for adolescents and young adults to express how they want to be cared for at the EoL and how they would like to be remembered (Five Wishes, 2023). These conversations may require specific language support, such as vocabulary to express wishes, and holistic team-based support.

Lead With Compassionate Curiosity

Be open to asking and learning about the patient's and family's wants, needs, perspectives, joys, and worries. Appreciate that your priorities, goals, and clinical agenda may not align with those of the patient and family. Be mindful of topics you know less about and demonstrate cultural humility, sensitivity, and compassion when inquiring about the preferences of the patient and those of the family. Use language patients and families will understand and enhance health literacy when necessary. Examples of statements and questions:

- It sounds like your family has a close bond. Tell me more about your special traditions.
- You mentioned not wanting Anton to hear the word "cancer." Can we think of other words to use when discussing his experience?

Establish Patient and Caregiver Understanding of Their Status

Many factors contribute to perspectives about serious illness, including age, cognition, culture, family dynamic, religion, community, and lived experience. Within families, parents and children may have different perspectives on the child's illness. Learning about the words used by family members when discussing disease, illness, interventions, and EoL concepts can inform supportive strategies and

approaches. To establish your understanding as a clinician, example phrases to use or adapt include:

- How would you describe your child's illness?
- What are the biggest challenges for Hassan right now?
- What does Isabelle understand about her illness?
- Are there certain words you or your child use to describe what is happening?
- Tell me more about how Alejandra has participated in conversations about her illness.

Calibrate Your Communication Style

Whether speaking to a child or their caregivers, it is essential to consider how you might pose questions, make statements, and gather information about a child's communication during a vulnerable experience. Some families appreciate levity and humor, while others may benefit from a more subtle and serious tone. These needs may change within the same family from day to day. Be open to adjusting your communication style and be attuned to your patients' and caregivers' needs.

- Be present; be prepared to listen more and talk less.
- Use sensitive language, but maintain clarity and avoid euphemisms.
- Follow the child's and family's lead. Do not assume; instead, ask.
- Appreciate that your idea of priorities and perspectives may differ from those of the child or family.
- Gauge readiness to discuss future-oriented goals. Use phrases like:
  - I would rather prepare you and your child for something your child may not need than have them need something they do not have.

- Learn about the child's personality and preferences. Use phrases such as:
  - Tell me about your child.
  - How would you describe Filip as a person?
  - What are their interests?
  - How does Makena like to receive medical information?
  - What matters most to you and your family when you think about Callum's communication?
  - What are you worried about?
  - Where does Sarah find her strength?
  - What brings Nasrin the most joy?
  - What are the things that are most important to Darius?

IMPLEMENTATION AND DEVELOPMENT OF ENGAGING TOOLS AND STRATEGIES

The implementation of strategies and continued SLP services in EoL care will look different for every child. Universally, the ability to remain flexible and prioritize dynamic reassessment and modification of needs, goals, and strategies is paramount to keeping each unique patient at the center of their care. Fried-Oken and Bardach (2005) describe a three-phase model for intervention in progressive illness, which is also applicable to care for children with life-limiting conditions. In the early phase of care, typically for individuals with baseline use of speech, intervention focuses on monitoring skills, preparation, and support through education and counseling. The second phase involves assessing skills and recommendations to support communication and implementation. In the late intervention phase, the SLP supports adaptation and accommodations to support functional life participation and uphold access to communication through EoL. At each phase, SLPs

target various areas of need in keeping with all the EoL considerations discussed earlier in this chapter. Primary domains for intervention are:

- Expressive communication
- Receptive communication
- Functional participation
- Maintaining relationships
- Building legacy

Timing of Speech-Language Pathology Intervention in Pediatric End-of-Life Care

A palliative approach to care starts at diagnosis for some young patients (Mack & Wolfe, 2006). Early intervention is imperative not only because a disease course may have a defined pattern of progression, but also because, in some cases, a slow, progressive decline may accelerate unexpectedly. For example, children with slow, progressive disease may experience acute neurological changes (e.g., stroke or hemorrhage), cardiac arrest, or respiratory arrest. When the SLP is involved early, communication and continuity of care are supported as the child's skills diminish with disease progression (Salt et al., 1999). Unfortunately, despite recommendations for early, proactive engagement, some children are not referred to an SLP until well into disease progression. Late referrals may also occur when families decline SLP involvement during the early phases of disease, for varied reasons such as concerns about cost, priorities, lack of knowledge about speech-language services, or being overwhelmed by the number and variety of medical appointments. However, it is never helpful to imply or describe why earlier referral could have been of benefit to a specific family. Strategies to encourage systems change are discussed in Chapter 2.

No matter the stage of disease progression at which the SLP first meets the child, even in the last days of life, communication assessment and intervention should be child focused, family oriented, and relationship centered. In the care of children in any setting, the family plays a unique role, which requires ongoing support from the SLP and the care team. Each child and family require continued focus on the child's physical, emotional, spiritual, and cognitive development (Krikheli et al., 2020).

SLP involvement throughout the EoL journey is closely tied to an individual child's unique needs and evolving status. Multiple variables, including alertness, medications, memory (Jackson et al., 1996); poor breath support and motor control for speech (Salt et al., 1999); word-finding difficulties, disease progression, fatigue, swelling, or sores of the mouth or airway, are considered, relative to the frequency of SLP involvement (Costello, 2000). Other factors that impact communication include the need for ventilator support, progressive loss of overall motor and/or motor speech skills, poor respiratory volume secondary to fatigue, the impact of medications for pain management, treatment of the underlying medical condition and/or sedation, and cognitive dampening. As a result, the need for communication intervention may be consistent or intermittent as the child nears EoL.

Allison, a 6-year-old female with DNA ligase IV deficiency, a rare autosomal recessive genetic disorder that causes combined immunodeficiency (Felgentreff et al., 2016), underwent a bone marrow transplant at a tertiary pediatric hospital center. Unfortunately, during her hospitalization, she developed a rare complication of post-transplant lymphoproliferative disorder (PTLD) and worsening respiratory distress. As Allison's respiratory status worsened, she was transferred to the intensive care unit (ICU) for initiation of an endotracheal tube and ventilation.

Over the course of several weeks, SLPs worked in collaboration with the patient's family, nurses, doctors, CLSs, music therapists, social workers, chaplains, and other health care team members to enhance Allison's communication and ability to control her environment and to participate in decision making while intubated. She effectively utilized voice-output communication aids (VOCAs) to gain attention, low-tech communication boards via multiple access methods for expressive communication, and a variety of unaided strategies to answer questions and to reflect her personality such as nonverbal eye rolls, pouted lips, smiles, and laughter. Even after removing the ventilator, Allison benefited from ongoing access to her AAC strategies as her voice and body remained weak. Over several months, her disease and respiratory decline progressed, ultimately requiring tracheostomy placement. At the same time, clinical care goals transitioned from curative to palliative care and focus on quality of life.

SLPs remained closely involved in Allison's care to ensure her communication needs, preferences, and social connections were maintained. Allison's mother requested support to initiate sign-supported speech of simple vocabulary because she had taught Allison some sign language as a very young child and thought sign language could provide Allison with increased assurance and comprehension. Access to expressive communication tools shifted from direct selection through pointing and eye gaze to partner-assisted auditory scanning as Allison had increased difficulty opening her eyes while awake. Nurses provided opportunities during all wakeful moments to promote Allison's participation through communication, inclusion in decision making and environmental control. During wakeful moments, her providers and family honored all unaided attempts to communication such as subtle head nods and changes in facial expression. A VOCA was initiated to ensure Allison could gain the attention of family members and clinical caregivers. When Allison's mother left the bedside to spend time with her other children for the weekend, a message was programmed using a previously recorded message, "Mommy, I love you!" Allison could initiate this message with a fist press on a switch and did so during assisted video calls with her mother over the weekend. Late in the weekend, Allison went into septic shock and passed away soon after her immediate and extended family returned to her side. Her last words were, "Mommy, I love you," played during an assisted video call the day prior to her death.

Allison's story exemplifies one we, as SLPs, hope never to encounter. When entering the field of pediatric speech and language pathology, we think of dynamic and language-rich experiences providing developmental and restorative practices to promote communication, feeding, social, play, and cognitive skills, but when a child requires EoL care, whether due to an expected disease trajectory or a sudden and acute change in status, SLPs must still support these exact needs for communication to promote quality of life and ultimately quality of death.

Eleven-year-old Yuto was asked what vocabulary he would want on a communication board if he ever struggled to speak. He immediately said, "Tell me a puppy story." When asked why he wanted a puppy story, he clarified that, when he is most stressed and most afraid, hearing stories about his puppies takes his attention away from the thing that is upsetting him.

Vocabulary Selection

Whenever possible, the SLP should engage the child and family in selecting the most appropriate vocabulary for communication of needs, social connectedness, coping, and personal self-expression (Figure 6–5). During this process, representations, including photos, symbols, or texts, are selected with the child to focus on comprehension of the representations. This selection step is particularly valuable when a child uses symbols for the first time to communicate.

Communication Strategies

As motor and sensory functions change, communication may be best supported using aided communication tools and alternative access options. While not all needs can be predicted, when children are invited to collaborate and can learn to understand and use eye pointing on communication boards, partner-assisted scanning, and other adapted communication strategies before they are needed, this early instruction and practice supports engagement later in the course of illness. In addition, identifying appropriate alternative access methods

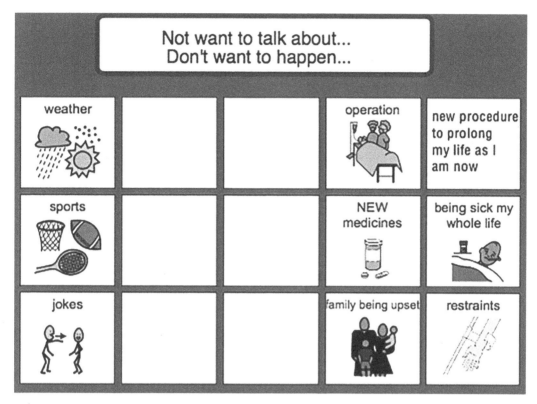

Figure 6–5. Example AAC board for child with a life-limiting illness.

through the dynamic feature-matched assessment ensures effective communication of important messages for medical care, comfort, and social connectedness.

Message Banking

Message banking is a clinical approach that allows people to record and store personally meaningful sounds, words, phrases, sentences, and/or stories using their own natural voice, inflection, and intonation. These messages are selected to reflect the identity and personality of the speaker. If needed, the recorded messages can be incorporated into the most appropriate technology to enhance communication and support the presentation of self because the emphasis is on the message's authenticity rather than specific words or intelligibility; rather, the intonation, phrasing, and emotional content are important (Costello, 2021).

Through message banking, a child can represent a more genuine self. Speaking in an authentic voice, even when using AAC, through proactive message banking can benefit the child, comfort family members, and allow the medical staff to relate to a child more richly than when a personal voice is not used (Costello, 2000). Tenderness, gratitude, humor, and sarcasm are more realistically communicated through personal voice. When appropriate, SLPs can counsel and educate patients and families on the benefits of message banking.

"My daughter's body looks so different. Her bright eyes, incessant chattering about anything and everything, and bouncing around the room with unstoppable energy are all gone. I know they are not coming back. The tubes, her weight loss, the change in her body composition, and her jaundiced color almost make me think it is not her. And then she presses the buttons on her communication device, and I hear 'I love you, Daddy' in her mischievous voice she used when she wanted to wrap me around her little finger, or I hear her whine, 'It's not fair!' or excitedly state with a giggle, 'I know I am your favorite child!' And my daughter is here with me. Everything looks different, but it is her voice, and I am reminded that I am sitting here with my little girl."

—Father of 7-year-old with acute lymphocytic leukemia (ALL)

Technoconnectedness

Technoconnectedness refers to using technology to retain social contacts, reduce isolation, and normalize communication (Fried Oken & Bardach, 2005). This may occur through accessible video calling, mobile technology, and other mediums (e.g., writing or dictating emails or letters, recording spoken or video messages). Collaboration with a CLS is extremely helpful to identify and implement bridging strategies with siblings, friends, and family members who may not be able to visit the child in-person. These strategies promote consistent language, explain complex concepts, and support the pediatric patient to optimize interactions, even when other important people are at a distance.

NORMALIZATION

Normalizing illness and the medical care experience will look different for each child. For some, this may entail access to favorite items and activities while in the hospital or in home care. For others, it may be passive or active participation in community events (e.g., school, religious entities or ceremonies, sporting experiences) in a manner aligned with the child's preferences and medical needs. For others, it is a consistent bedtime story or phone call with a grandparent. Establishing or preserving a daily routine can promote a sense of normalcy. Routines also allow for anticipation of upcoming tasks or special activities. Children often benefit from visual schedules to enhance their understanding of what is next, especially when faced with a changing body and mind.

Maintaining Social Connectedness and Emotional Closeness

Family and peer relationships are significant to children. Serious illness creates some social and physical barriers to these friendships and connections. For families, the loss of social connectedness with a child may be a leading contributor to grief. However, AAC strategies may support continued connectedness and maintain special social closeness. In one instance, a mother reported that one of her most special connections with her 4-year-old son was singing "You Are My Sunshine" together. As his speaking ability became more intermittent, the SLP recorded him singing the song on a single-switch voice-output aid. In subsequent weeks, he was able to select the switch and activate his own voice to sing along with his mother.

"Looking at Matthias, um, end-of-life stage, and I know eventually what that means, but don't take the communication away from me just yet. That's all we have left. And what I find with Mattie through most of his day is that it's no longer 'I have to go pee,' 'Get me water,' or 'I want to watch TV.' It's the 'You're my sweetie pie,' 'You're my heart,' 'I love you,' or 'Get your big head out of my way.' I find that it is what makes him happy and it makes us still laugh because that's who he is. I feel that if he loses his communication, I am losing Mattie because that is what makes us who we are as people. It is how we comfort each other, make each other laugh, and stay connected. My learning experience is that people have to understand how crucial it is to have that voice. For me, the mother of a child with a ter-minal illness, these are wonderful things. I feel so empty when I cannot connect with Mattie. It is sad, very sad. Because that is my whole way of connecting. He is a child who could always speak, and when it is diminished, sometimes it is so hard, but he can't say everything he wants back. So, to have the recordings of his little 'isms' and even his sarcasm and insults, it brings us both great comfort. We can still be close, and he can still connect with others on his terms. Every speech pathologist or any staff in palliative care must know that recording a voice before losing it is the greatest gift you can give someone who is dying. Moreover, you can give loved ones the greatest gift after their child is gone. It may sound crazy, but it gives me hope; hope that I will not lose all of him, even when he's gone."

—Mother of Matthias, age 12 years with juvenile Huntington's disease

Support for Reflection of Positive Life Events

As children experience more significant impacts of disease, it is common to note a shift in their communication interests. A child initially focused on autonomy, control, and self-determination may become more interested in sharing and hearing stories about enjoyable experiences and life events as significant loss of motor and speech skills occurs.

When David first lost his ability to speak, he remained interested in directing the behavior of others and self-advocating with messages such as "no," "stop," and "go away"; requesting food (that he could not eat); choosing games; and selecting television programs. The SLP created a multipage communication notebook for him to support this communication. As his disease progressed, David's mother reported that he appeared more interested in looking through photos on her smartphone. This prompted her to bring family photo albums to the hospital. The SLP introduced a talking photo album and David selected photos from the family photo album to be included. With his parents helping co-construct messages as David pointed to salient features in a photo (e.g., balloons, a cake, an inflatable pool float), a story was recorded to correspond to each of the photos in the talking photo album. David's mother reported that for the last 2 weeks of his life, David was solely interested in someone sitting with him so he could "tell the story" of each photo. He particularly enjoyed it when his communication partner added more details, often leading to David and his family laughing as they reminisced. When his strength diminished and he could no longer activate the message, David would point to a photo to direct his communication partner to activate the recorded message.

Supporting Expression of Legacy

Legacy is defined as a "process of leaving something behind," which can include "one's belongings, one's memories, one's values, and even one's body" (Hunter & Rowles, 2005). Building a legacy can occur at any point in a child's life and illness trajectory. It is about making connections and sharing precious moments with the special people in your life (Griffith, 2011). Often, patients and families participate in projects and activities with the intent to build a legacy, which can be accomplished in many ways. The SLP may work toward this aim with the patient, family, and interprofessional team. For children who have reduced use of natural speech and are using AAC strategies, SLPs can support the design and creation of tools that assist participation in and direction of these activities. For example, a teenager worked with her SLP and music therapist to record her heartbeat and overlaid it with a favorite song encapsulated in a recorder in a teddy bear. Other legacy activities previously noted in this chapter include message banking, recording songs, creating a photo album, and compiling audio or video recordings from loved ones to the patient for passive listening.

Creating Social Stories or Books

Social stories and person-centered narratives are common ways to enhance comprehension of abstract concepts. Children approaching EoL may benefit from using stories to understand processes, events, and expectations. Stories may facilitate difficult conversations in a child-focused, simple, and developmentally appropriate way.

Case Study: Social Story

Joey, a 5-year-old boy with chromosome 18q deletion syndrome, experienced multisystem end-organ failure in complex cancer management. After 6 weeks in the pediatric intensive care unit, Joey's heart stopped. After the cardiac arrest his overall prognosis worsened. Joey communicated feelings of "worry" and "being scared" to nurses while intubated using a basic communication board, and the ICU team requested SLP services for additional support. In conversation with the SLP, social worker, and CLS, Joey's mother told the providers through tears that Joey "just doesn't understand what is happening to him." His mother requested help explaining what was happening to help alleviate Joey's feelings of worry and fear. The SLP and CLS, along with Joey's mom, created a developmentally appropriate social story. The story used relevant patient photographs and language consistent with that used by his mom and care team to support comprehension of his health status and ways he might cope with that information. The story was simplified as Joey became sleepier and more unstable. Care team and family members continued to read Joey his story as care goals shifted to comfort care and do not resuscitate (DNR)/do not intubate (DNI) orders were put in place. The story helped to reduce fear and anxiety for Joey and members of his family also found comfort in the story.

Excerpts from Joey's social story:

- Kids come to the hospital for many different reasons.
- You came to the hospital because your body was very sick. The doctors and nurses have been helping your body get better, but your body is still so, so, so sick.
- The doctors and nurses are working very hard to help your body. But, even with all the medicine and special help, your body isn't getting better.
- Right now, the doctors and nurses are making sure your body stays comfortable.
- They are here all day and all night to keep you safe. You can let them know if you feel worried or uncomfortable.
- Being sick at the hospital might make you feel lots of feelings. Any way you are feeling is OK. If you are ever feeling scared or worried, you can hold Mom's hand and think about your favorite things, like fire trucks and your family!
- You could remember: "Mom is always with me and stays at the hospital all day and night. She makes sure I have company and I'm safe, just like the nurses."
- Even if your body is very sick, you are still brave, fun, and kind.
- Everyone is so proud of you!

CONCLUSION

The SLP is critical in the care of a child with a life-limiting illness. As medical, motor, cognitive, and sensory status each change throughout the illness, the dynamic engagement of the SLP is critical to support participation in many powerful themes ranging from preserving childhood experiences through play and social engagement to maintaining social connectedness and expression of legacy. Integration of AAC through communication planning at early phases of illness via message banking, and evolving tools and strategies over time, should be carefully considered through dynamic assessment and reassessment of a child's unique needs and desires. Early engagement is valuable, when possible, because it allows for ongoing support of the child and family as collaborative partners in system and strategy selection, implementation, and development.

A NOTE TO THE READER ON SELF-CARE

"Today, I said goodbye to a patient and his parents. It was a hard day."

I first met Isaac 2.5 years ago in our ICU following an emergency resection of a brain tumor. He was diagnosed with medulloblastoma, and 2 days postoperatively, Isaac stopped speaking and began a difficult and long journey recovering from cerebellar mutism syndrome (also known as posterior fossa syndrome). Over a period of months, Isaac and I spent a lot of time together working on his communication. We spent almost every weekday using various AAC tools and strategies, which naturally evolved with his recovery. Every day that I worked with Isaac, I learned something new about him from his personality, interests, humor, and talents, all while he was unable to speak and barely able to move. I prioritized a "life participation approach" by focusing on his interests, motivations, personality traits, and priorities jointly with his parents and care team members. I started to cotreat with members of our Child Life Program and began to witness all the beautiful attributes of this 9-year-old boy come to life. I also witnessed him regain the use of speech over time, which allowed him and his parents to reflect on the incredible benefits of AAC during a time of need.

When Isaac's cancer relapsed a few months ago, he began to experience changes in his physical and mental status all over again. His speech production and cognition fluctuated throughout the day. The medical team asked me to consult again a couple of weeks before he passed, this time to support his cognitive/communication skills as he was dying. His final weeks were a challenge, as his parents felt they were slowly losing pieces of their son. So, I listened a lot. We discussed supportive strategies and ways to enhance his communication, connection, and control in the face of an undetermined timeline. The next day, I spent an hour with Isaac, letting him control the conversation the entire time and employing these strategies subtly. His parents said it was the most he had talked in over a week. They thanked me for giving them and Isaac that moment. During that conversation, Isaac gave me a gift to give my children, and I made a promise to give one in return. "Well, you don't have to do that. But that is nice of you," he told me.

Today, Isaac has not woken up. But I kept my promise and gave his parents his gift. We cried, hugged, and thanked each other for everything the other had done. We shared memories of Isaac and reflected on his spirit and resilience. We laughed through tears and told each other to be good. Then I walked down to my office and allowed myself to cry.

We cannot tell you how to care for yourself before, during, or after the loss of a patient. The death of a child is incredibly challenging; it may feel strange to think about taking care of yourself after caring for a dying child. However, burnout and compassion fatigue are common and, frankly, are expected if you do not find ways to incorporate self-care and balance. You may still feel lots of feelings, and that is OK. However, there are some ways to help yourself heal and recover when grieving the death of a pediatric patient:

- Participate in bereavement debriefing sessions with colleagues if they are offered. Share stories and memories with others who also cared for your patients. You will be amazed at how these acts of sharing can provide comfort. You may even learn things you did not know about the patient from them, enriching your memory.
- Write a letter to the family. Our PPC team gathered feedback from families and found they greatly appreciate handwritten notes from care providers. Remind them of a fond memory of their child that is personal and genuine. They will appreciate hearing from you and you will likely find comfort and closure in writing to them.
- Engage in supportive offerings through your work. At our institution, we have an annual ceremony for families who have lost a child who had been cared for at our institution. There,

we can reconnect with and support the families we have met. We also have bereavement counselors and champions on every unit who support staff after a patient has passed.

- Do something for you. Eat a piece of chocolate, go for a run, engage in a hobby, or watch a movie. Do something that brings you joy.
- Take a break if you need it. This can mean going for a walk during lunch or allowing yourself to take a day (or

days) off work. Give yourself permission to pause and acknowledge your grief.

Above all, remember that you have made a difference. Isaac's parents always used to tell me, "We wish we never *had* to meet you, but we're so grateful that we did." I'm forever grateful to all the children I've met and the families who allowed me to help care for them.

—Rachel

"I will love my son, with every fiber of my being for every second I have him with me and continue to memorize every detail of how he feels in my arms. I know that I need to store up these memories because this glimpse into the future is a reminder to me that our time on this earth is fleeting, and we need to make it count." —Randell, 2017

REFERENCES

Adistie, F., Lumbantobing, V. B., & Maryam, N. N. A. (2020). The needs of children with terminal illness: A qualitative study. *Child Care in Practice, 26*(3), 257–271.

American Academy of Pediatrics. (2016). Informed consent in decision-making in pediatric practice. *Pediatrics, 138*(2), e1484–1491. https://doi.org/10.1542/peds.2016-1484

Association of Child Life Professionals. (2023). *The child life profession.* https://www.childlife.org/the-child-life-profession

Berlin, A. (2017). Goals of care and end of life in the ICU. *Surgical Clinics, 97*(6), 1275–1290.

Brewer, J. (2020, April 22). *Helping your kids face their uncertainty.* Elemental. https://elemental.medium.com/helping-your-kids-face-their-uncertainty-7d44295ee61b

Brewster, A. B. (1982). Chronically ill hospitalized children's concepts of their illness. *Pediatrics, 69*(3), 355–362.

Brinkman-Stoppelenburg, A., Rietjens, J. A., & van der Heide, A. (2014). The effects of advance care planning on end-of-life care: A systematic review. *Palliative Medicine, 28*(8), 1000–1025. https://doi.org/10.1177/0269216314526272

Center to Advance Palliative Care. (2019). *America's care of serious illness: 2019 state-by-state report card on access to palliative care in our nation's hospitals.* Center to Advance Palliative Care and the National Palliative Care Research Center. https://reportcard.capc.org/

Chiu, A. T. G., Wong, S. S. N., Wong, N. W. T., Wong, W. H. S., Tso, W. W. Y., & Fung, C. W. (2022). Quality of life and symptom burden in children with neurodegenerative diseases: Using PedsQL and SProND, a new symptom-based scale. *Orphanet Journal of Rare Diseases, 17*, 334. https://doi.org/10.1186/s13023-022-02485-5

Cohen, E., Kuo, D., Agrawal, R., Berry, J., Bhagat, S., Simon. T., & Srivastava, R. (2011). Children with medical complexity: An emerging population for clinical and research initiatives. *Pediatrics, 127*(3), 529–538. https://doi.org/10.1542/peds.2010-0910

Costello, J. (2000). AAC intervention in the intensive care unit: The Children's Hospital Boston model. *Augmentative and Alternative Commu-*

nication, *16*(3), 137–153. https://www.doi.org/10.1080/07434610012331279004

Costello, J. (2009). Last words, last connections: How augmentative communication can support children facing end of life. *The ASHA Leader, 14*(16), 8–11. https://www.doi.org/10.1044/leader.FTR2.14162009.8

Costello, J. M., Patak, L., & Pritchard, J. (2010). Communication vulnerable patients in the pediatric ICU: Enhancing care through augmentative and alternative communication. *Journal of Pediatric Rehabilitation Medicine, 3*(4), 289–301. https://www.doi.org/10.3233/PRM-2010-0140

Costello, J., & Smith, M. (2021). The BCH message banking process, voice banking, and double-dipping. *Augmentative and Alternative Communication, 37*(4), 241–250. https://www.doi.org/10.1080/07434618.2021.2021554

Eiser, C. (1985). Changes in understanding of illness as the child grows. *Archives of Disease in Childhood, 60*(5), 489–492.

Eissler, R. S., Kriss, M., & Solnitt, A. J. (1977). *Physical illness and handicap in childhood.* Yale University Press.

Felgentreff, K., Baxi, S. N., Lee, Y. N., Dobbs, K., Henderson, L. A., Csomos, K., . . . Notarangelo, L. D. (2016). Ligase-4 deficiency causes distinctive immune abnormalities in asymptomatic individuals. *Journal of Clinical Immunology, 36*(4), 341–353. https://doi.org/10.1007/s10875-016-0266-5

Five Wishes. (2023). *My wishes and voicing my choices.* https://www.fivewishes.org/for-myself/

Fried-Oken, M., & Bardach, L. (2005). End-of-life issues for people who use AAC. *Perspectives on Augmentative and Alternative Communication, 14*(3), 15–19.

Gilboa, S. M., Devine, O. J., Kucik, J. E., Oster, M. E., Riehle-Colarusso, T., Nembhard, W. N., . . . Marelli, A. J. (2016). Congenital heart defects in the United States: Estimating the magnitude of the affected population in 2010. *Circulation, 134*(2), 101–109. https://doi.org/10.1161/CIRCULATIONAHA.115.019307

Gillis, J., & Loughlan, P. (2007). Not just small adults: The metaphors of paediatrics. *Archives of Disease in Childhood, 92*(11), 946–947.

Griffith, W. (2011, July 26). *Making memories last: The art of legacy work.* MD Anderson Cancer Center. https://www.mdanderson.org/cancerwise/making-memories-last-the-art-of-legacy-work.h00-158673423.html

Hawksley, R., Ludlow, F., Buttimer, H., & Bloch, S. (2017). Communication disorders in palliative care: Investigating the views, attitudes and beliefs of speech and language therapists. *International Journal of Palliative Nursing, 23*(11), 543–551. https://doi.org/10.12968/ijpn.2017.23.11.543

Himebauch, A., Arnold, R. M., & May, C. (2008). Grief in children and developmental concepts of death #138. *Journal of Palliative Medicine, 11*(2), 242–244.

Himelstein, B. P. (2006). Palliative care for infants, children, adolescents, and their families. *Journal of Palliative Care Medicine, 9*(1), 163–181. http://doi.org/10.1089/jpm.2006.9.163

Hunter, E., & Rowles, G. (2005). Leaving a legacy: Toward a typology. *Journal of Aging Studies, 19*, 327–347.

Jackson, P., Robbins, M., & Frankel, S. (1996). Communication impediments in a group of hospice patients. *Medicine, 10*, 79–80.

Johnson, E., Bornman, J., & Tonsing, M. (2016). An exploration of pain-related vocabulary: Implications for AAC use with children. *Augmentative and Alternative Communication, 32*(4), 249–260.

Krikheli, L., Erickson, S., Carey, L. B., Carey-Sargeant, C. L., & Mathisen, B. A. (2020). Perspectives of speech and language therapists in paediatric palliative care: An international exploratory study. *International Journal of Language & Communication Disorders, 55*(4), 558–572.

Krikheli, L., Erickson, S., Carey, L. B., Carey-Sargeant, C. L., & Mathisen, B. A. (2021). Speech-language pathologists in pediatric palliative care: An international study of perceptions and experiences. *American Journal of Speech-Language Pathology, 30*(1), 150–168. https://doi.org/10.1044/2020_AJSLP-20-00090

Lerwick, J. L. (2016). Minimizing pediatric healthcare-induced anxiety and trauma. *World Journal of Clinical Pediatrics, 5*(2), 143.

Lyman, J., Maurer, S., Baker, J., & Kane, J. (2008, November). *Communicating with the dying child* [Paper presentation]. Meeting of the 19th World Congress of Children's Hospice International, San Francisco, CA, United States.

Mack, J. W., & Wolfe, J. (2006). Early integration of pediatric palliative care: For some children, palliative care starts at diagnosis. *Current Opinion in Pediatrics, 18*(1), 10–14. https://doi.org/10.1097/01.mop.0000193266.86129.47

Piaget, J. (1951). *Play, dreams and imitation in childhood*. Routledge. https://doi.org/10.4324/9781315009698

Pollens, R. (2020). Facilitating client ability to communicate in palliative end-of-life care: Impact of speech-language pathologists. *Topics in Language Disorders, 40*(3), 264–277. https://doi.org/10.1097/TLD.0000000000000220

Randell, I. (2017). *Anticipatory grief*. Complex Child. https://complexchild.org/articles/2017-articles/march/anticipatory-grief/

Salt, N., Dasies, S., & Wilkinson, S. (1999). The contribution of speech and language therapy to palliative care. *European Journal of Palliative Care, 6*(4), 126–129.

Sansom-Daly, U. M., Wakefield, C. E., Patterson, P., Cohn, R. J., Rosenberg, A. R., Wiener, L., & Fardell, J. E. (2020). End-of-life communication needs for adolescents and young adults with cancer: Recommendations for research and practice. *Journal of Adolescent and Young Adult Oncology, 9*(2), 157–165. https://doi.org/10.1089/jayao.2019.0084

Shane, H., & J. Costello (1994, November). *Augmentative communication assessment and the feature matching process*. American Speech Language Hearing Association Annual Convention, New Orleans, LA, United States.

Snaman, J. M., Torres, C., Duffy, B., Levine, D. R., Gibson, D. V., & Baker, J. N. (2016). Parental perspectives of communication at the end of life at a pediatric oncology institution. *Journal of Palliative Medicine, 19*(3), 326–332. https://doi.org/10.1089/jpm.2015.0253

Sue, K., Mazzotta, P., & Grier, E. (2019). Palliative care for patients with communication and cognitive difficulties. *Canadian Family Physician, 65*(Suppl. 1), S19–S24. https://www.ncbi.nlm.nih.gov/pmc/articles/PMC6501717/

University of California San Diego. (2020). *Psychosocial needs of the dying child*. https://myhealth.ucsd.edu/RelatedItems/90,P03055

Wolfelt, A. (2007). *Helping a child who is dying*. Center for Loss and Life Transition. https://www.centerforloss.com/bookstore/helping-a-child-who-is-dying-100/

Wong-Baker FACES Foundation. (n.d.). *Wong-Baker FACES Pain Rating Scale*. https://wongbakerfaces.org/

World Health Organization Expert Committee on Cancer Pain Relief and Active Support Care. (1990). Cancer pain relief and palliative care: Report of a WHO expert committee. *World Health Organization Technical Report Series, 804*, 1–75.

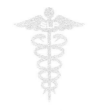

APPENDIX A

Resources to Support Teaching About Death, Dying, and End-of-Life Care

Amanda Stead and Jordan Tinsley

TEACHING ABOUT DEATH, DYING, AND END-OF-LIFE CARE

Communication is essential for people nearing the end of life (EoL). Speech-language pathologists (SLPs) play a critical role in the care of patients with life-limiting conditions as advocates for effective communication and access to quality-of-life-enhancing activities including eating and drinking. Understanding the SLP's roles and responsibilities with this patient population goes beyond assessment and treatment of individual impairments. Effective engagement in EoL care includes awareness of individual biases and fears associated with the topics of death and dying, the goals of palliative care, and knowledge of the systems for care delivery through medical, long-term, palliative, and hospice care.

The concepts of a palliative care approach apply to the work of SLPs across settings. Very few academic programs prepare students for the death of a patient (client, resident, or student), yet patients die in acute care, reha-

bilitation, long-term care, and home health settings. Patients with life-limiting conditions are routinely seen in outpatient clinics and in educational settings. All SLPs, regardless of their intended career path, benefit from the opportunity to learn about and reflect on EoL care.

By exposing students to comprehensive content related to EoL care, programs can improve patient outcomes and professional confidence and reduce career burnout. Learner outcomes and competency goals for educating SLP students should include the following:

- Recognize one's attitudes, feelings, values, and expectations about death and the role of individual, cultural, religious, and spiritual diversity bound to these beliefs and customs.
- Demonstrate respect for the patient's preferences, values, and goals throughout the EoL trajectory.
- Understand the role of the SLP within an interdisciplinary team context to implement effective EoL care.

- Conduct assessments and develop intervention goals that integrate patients' physical, psychological, social, and spiritual needs.
- Assist the patient, family, colleagues, and oneself to cope with suffering grief, loss, and bereavement. (Rivers et al., 2009)

While it would be optimal to build a freestanding course with comprehensive coverage of palliative and EoL care, we recognize that most graduate programs simply cannot accommodate the addition of new coursework. In many ways, the integration of EoL care across the curriculum normalizes the care of patients with life-limiting conditions as an expected part of the work of the SLP. No one course instructor will be able to integrate all the learning outcomes into one course. However, with collaboration across courses, these objectives could be met across the graduate curriculum.

Table A–1 provides suggested course objectives, subobjectives, activities, and assignments that course instructors can use or modify to integrate into an existing course. These constructs apply in every area of practice and could be integrated anywhere in the curriculum, but may be particularly relevant in coursework focused on counseling, professionalism and ethics, dysphagia, progressive neurologic disorders, aphasia, cognitive communication disorders, and/or aging. Palliative and EoL care examples can also be used in interprofessional education experiences.

Table A–1. Suggested Course Objectives, Subobjectives, and Activities for Teaching Content in End-of-Life Care

Objectives	Activities and Assessment Examples
Main objective: • Explore the end-of-life (EoL) care experience in a human-centered context Subobjectives: • Encounter and/or examine the student's personal relationship to death and dying and how their lived experience may impact their work • Develop and practice therapeutic communication for use in EoL care • Consider aspects of grief, loss, and bereavement of patients and families • Discuss and consider the experience of death and dying on clinicians	Read: • Chapter 1 of this text • Morgan, D., Rawlings, D., Button, E., & Tieman, J. (2019). Allied health clinicians' understanding of palliative care as it relates to patients, caregivers, and health clinicians: A cross-sectional survey. *Journal of Allied Health, 48*(2), 127–133. • Sedig, L. K., Spruit, J. L., Paul, T. K., Cousino, M. K., Pituch, K., & Hutchinson, R. (2020). Experiences at the end of life from the perspective of bereaved parents: Results of a qualitative focus group study. *American Journal of Hospice and Palliative Medicine, 37*(6), 424–432. Assignment: Explore the Conversation Project website (www.conversationproject.org) and complete the starter kit. Respond to discussion forum questions: 1. While exploring the Conversation Project website, what information was new to you or caused you to think about something previously unconsidered? 2. What, if any, feelings or thoughts did you have while completing your own kit? 3. What is your current understanding of your future professional role in EoL care? Watch: The documentary *Extremis* (https://www.netflix.com/title/80106307). Please reflect on the following questions and submit them for your weekly assignment. 1. What were your initial thoughts on the documentary? 2. How were the doctors and staff communicating about issues of decision making? Were there differences in their professional communication? What do you believe their viewpoints were? 3. When you think about EoL decisions for patients, what is the difference between your viewpoint (what you would do) and what you communicate to patients? 4. What strategies do you think you are most likely to use? 5. What risks are involved in the way we communicate these options and our own opinions?

continues

Table A–1. *continued*

Objectives	Activities and Assessment Examples

Main Objective:
 	
• Understand the biology of death and health systems aspects of end-of-life (EoL) care
 	
Subobjectives:
 	
• Understand expected physiological changes at the EoL
 	
• Differentiate between palliative care and hospice care
 	
• Consider the implications of interventions typically used at the EoL
	Read:
	
	• Chapter 1 of this text
	• Dunn, G. P., & Milch, R. A. (2002). Is this a bad day, or one of the last days? How to recognize and respond to approaching demise. *Journal of the American College of Surgeons*, *195*(6), 879–887.
	• Hospice Foundation of America. (n.d.). *Signs of approaching death*. https://hospicefoundation.org/Hospice-Care/Signs-of-Approaching-Death
	• Shalev, A., Phongtankuel, V., Kozlov, E., Shen, M. J., Adelman, R. D., & Reid, M. C. (2018). Awareness and misperceptions of hospice and palliative care: A population-based survey study. *The American Journal of Hospice & Palliative Care*, *35*(3), 431–439. https://doi.org/10.1177/1049909117715215
	
	Watch: "At What Moment Are You Dead?" https://www.youtube.com/watch?v=5c6C3rHOdf8
	
	Assignment: Given what you know about the symptoms accompanying the final weeks/days of someone's life, please answer the following questions:
	
	1. Choose one of the primary signs/symptoms (breathing issues, pain, emotional distress, food/drink intake, mobility) of approaching death and describe how your professional role intersects with that symptom's management.
	  a. What is your professional role in the general care of this symptom (think about your scope of practice)?
	  b. How can you imagine you could support the patient or family with managing this symptom near the EoL?
	2. Why is it essential to manage this particular symptom, and how does this contribute to quality care and a positive dying experience?
	
	Watch: The documentary *End Game* (https://www.netflix.com/title/80210691) and respond to the following questions in a reflection paper.
	
	1. What are the goals of hospice and what are the challenges associated with meeting these goals?
	2. Reflect on how watching this documentary made you feel and what you were thinking about while watching it.

Table A–1. *continued*

Objectives	Activities and Assessment Examples

Main Objective:
 	
• Consider legal and ethical issues in EoL care
 	
Subobjectives:
 	
• Discuss specific ethical and legal issues
 	
• Differentiate capacity from competency and apply these constructs to case-based scenarios
 	
• Describe key elements of EoL documentation
	Read:
	
	• Chapter 3 of this text
	
	• Leo, R. J. (1999). Competency and the capacity to make treatment decisions: A primer for primary care physicians. *Primary Care Companion to the Journal of Clinical Psychiatry, 1*(5), 131–141. https://doi.org/10.4088/pcc.v01n0501
	
	• Stead, A., & McDonnell, C. (2015). Discussing end-of-life care: An opportunity. *Perspectives on Gerontology, 20*(1), 12–15.
	
	Listen: "The Bitter End" from Radiolab: https://www.radiolab.org/episodes/262588-bitter-end
	
	Assignment: Consider a case study related to clinical decision-making capacity and legal competence.
	
	Example Case:
	
	Mrs. Tremblay has been admitted to the hospital following a fall at home. She is 85 years old and lives on her own. Until now, she has managed independently with support from her neighbors and her daughter, who lives 50 miles away. The fall resulted in a marked reduction in mobility. She is unable to bear weight and requires full support with her personal care needs. At times Mrs. Tremblay is confused about where she is and what happened to her. Mrs. Tremblay has been assessed by a physiotherapist, who recommends nursing home placement to provide adequate assistance with physical care needs. Mrs. Tremblay's daughter supports this recommendation as she feels she would not be able to offer her mother the support she needs if she returned home. However, at this stage, a social worker has not assessed Mrs. Tremblay, and there is the potential for her needs to be met at home through home health and other support systems. Mrs. Tremblay has stated that she does not want to go into a nursing home.
	
	1. What are the issues to consider related to this patient's discharge plan?
	
	2. Do you think Mrs. Tremblay has the capacity to make this decision?
	   a. If you do, why?
	   b. If not, why not, and how have you reached this decision?
	
	3. What other concerns might you have about Mrs. Tremblay's situation and how might you address these?
	
	4. Who should be involved in this decision?

continues

Table A–1. *continued*

Objectives	Activities and Assessment Examples
Main Objective: • Explore and articulate professional roles and responsibilities	Read: • Chapter 2 of this text • Pollens, R. (2020). Facilitating client ability to communicate in palliative end-of-life care: Impact of speech-language pathologists. *Topics in Language Disorders*, 40(3), 264–277.
Subobjectives: • Demonstrate a baseline understanding of the roles and responsibilities of different allied health professionals in the care and treatment of people with life-limiting illness and at the EoL • Consider roles and responsibilities of the SLP special populations	Assignment: • Identify and annotate at least three peer-reviewed articles related to the roles and responsibilities of allied health professionals in EoL care. • In the discussion forum, describe what you learned about your professional role in palliative or EoL care. • Identify another allied health discipline and write a brief post about how you could partner with that discipline to improve the quality of care for patients with life-limiting conditions or nearing the EoL. Watch: "What Matters at the End" https://www.ted.com/talks/bj_miller_what_really_matters_at_the_end_of_life?language=en Create: Develop an infographic that educates colleagues from your discipline about one crucial aspect of EoL care you believe is relevant to high quality practice. Use the website https://piktochart.com/ to help you create the infographic. Your infographic should include the following: • Vibrant visuals • At least three primary, evidenced-based references • A clear title and orientation to the topic • Clear takeaway message(s) Assignment: In addition to creating the infographic, submit a reflective paper that addresses the following questions related to your infographic. 1. Why is this infographic helpful to your colleagues? Could it be helpful to other audiences? 2. What contexts do you think would be most helpful for sharing this information (e.g., pinned to a bulletin board, available at the patient's bedside, presented in a class, emailed to colleagues)? 3. Write a short paragraph about content you decided to exclude and why you opted to leave it out or chose to emphasize other information. 4. List all references used to construct your infographic.

SUGGESTED ACTIVITY FOR DYSPHAGIA COURSE

Within the dysphagia curriculum, issues related to risks, comfort care, saliva management, oral care, and service delivery are considered. Examples should include how to plan management for a patient who is not going to get better, palliative care pathways, and to introduce palliative care concepts (Pascoe et al., 2018). This activity can be structured as a simulation (using actors to serve as the patient's surrogate decision maker and any other members of the care team present in the care conference) or as an in-class role-play.

Assigned Readings

Chapters 3 and 5 of this text supplemented by one or more of the following:

- Askren, A. N., & Kershner, M. (2020). Eating, drinking, and comfort at end-of-life: Promoting a quality of death. *Perspectives of the ASHA Special Interest Groups*, 5(4), 1015–1020.
- Leslie, P., & Coyle, J. (2010). Complex decisions involving gastrostomy feeding tubes: When you're never right or wrong. *Perspectives on Gerontology*, 15(2), 42–47.
- Vitale, C. A., Berkman, C. S., Monteleoni, C., & Ahronheim, J. C. (2011). Tube feeding in patients with advanced dementia: Knowledge and practice of speech-language pathologists. *Journal of Pain and Symptom Management*, 42(3), 366–378.

Class Activity: Instructions for Students

The purpose of the activity is to allow you to demonstrate your ability to navigate a patient care conference. You will provide emotional support in the context of a conversation with a family member. You should be able to explain your roles and responsibilities in the care of a person near the EoL and the evidence related to appropriate care based on patient status. At the end of the session, you should be able to:

- Navigate a care conference with a family and provide emotional support
- Explain the roles and responsibilities of SLPs in the care of a person near the EoL
- Explain the evidence related to appropriate care based on patient status
- Reflect on efficacy of the communication and identify what you would modify in future clinical contexts

Background Information Provided to Students Before the Care Conference

SLPs work as part of an interdisciplinary team that cares for those near the EoL. You will serve as the SLP in a conversation with another member of the interdisciplinary team and a family member of a patient. This conversation will take place in the context of a care conference. The purpose of the care conference is to discuss the treatment plan for a patient with late-stage dementia who is nearing EoL.

The patient is not eating well and has been losing weight. The patient does not have any advance medical orders. This means the team would run a full-code cardiopulmonary resuscitation if the patient's heart stops. The patient named an adult child as a surrogate decision maker but did not provide any specific preferences through a living will. The patient's family is concerned about weight loss and have asked about whether the team is considering tube feeding.

As the lead SLP, you must use your clinical judgment and consider the patient's values, well-being, and desired outcomes when supporting the family through this conversation and decision making. Your role is to balance the complex factors of this case and present current evidence regarding the use of artificially administered nutrition/hydration for patients with advanced dementia while simultaneously providing counseling to the family member.

Patient Information

Emilija Matas is an 81-year-old female with advanced Alzheimer's dementia (Stage 7 on the Global Deterioration Scale). Mrs. Matas currently resides in the Fieldstone Memory Care facility. Over the past year, caregivers at the facility have observed a gradual decline in function and level of independence. At this time, Mrs. Matas needs assistance for all activities of daily living. Mrs. Matas currently consumes regular food and drink textures, with some assistance at each meal. Caregivers have observed decreased intake in the past month (<50% of each meal), leading to unintentional weight loss. More recently, caregivers

have noticed increased swallowing difficulty and coughing episodes during meals, which yielded a referral for speech-language services related to dysphagia.

Instructions

If structured as a role-play, the activity takes place in two rounds (approximately 5 minutes each). First, divide students into pairs. One student plays the role of the SLP, and the other plays the role of the adult child. Provide the student acting as the adult child with the Round 1 prompts listed in Table A–2 and begin the timer for 5 minutes. Following Round 1, ask the students to switch roles and provide the new adult child with the second round of prompts. Following another 5 minutes of role playing, debrief the students about what they learned from the experience, what successes they had in communication, what challenges they faced, and how they will navigate these encounters in the future.

Table A–2. Prompts for the Adult Child in a Role-Play Activity (or Standardized Patient Activity) in Decision Making About Artificially Administered Nutrition and Hydration

Round 1 prompts	• "I just saw my mom last week, and it seemed like things were going well." • "If you are a speech therapist, why are you working on my mom's eating?" • "Will my mom's eating get better?" • "How long has this been going on? And what does aspiration mean?" • "So basically, you are saying that my mom will continue to lose weight and that any food and drink she eats has a chance to go down to her lungs?" • "I am not sure about the feeding tube. My mom loves to eat or used to anyway."
Round 2 prompts	• "What are the possible options?" • "Are there any other options?" • "Is there anything I can do to help my mom?" • "Why isn't a feeding tube a good option for her?" • "My mom loves to eat. Is there any way we can make it easier?" • "If I were to decide on comfort feeding, what would that look like?"

SUGGESTED ACTIVITY FOR ALTERNATIVE AUGMENTATIVE COMMUNICATION (AAC), APHASIA, MOTOR SPEECH, OR COGNITIVE/ COMMUNICATION COURSE

Communication and cognitive impairments can place patients at risk for diminished autonomy, socialization, and participation. Patients with communication or cognitive barriers are at risk of exclusion from medical decision making based on assumptions that they lack capacity for decision making. Augmentative and alternative communication (AAC) can support patients' communication, participation in decision making, and social engagement. AAC can also support the psychological and spiritual aspects of EoL care (Leslie & Broll, 2022; Pollens, 2020; Stead, 2022).

Assigned Readings

- Chapters 2 and 4 of this text
- Pollens, R. (2020). Facilitating client ability to communicate in palliative end-of-life care. *Topics in Language Disorders*, 40(3), 264–277. https://10.1097/ TLD.0000000000000220
- Stead, A. (2022). End-of-life care for adults. In N. Hall, J. Juengling-Sudkamp, M. L. Gutmann, & E. R. Cohn (Eds.), *Fundamentals in AAC: A case-based approach to enhancing communication.* Plural Publishing.

Class Activity or Assignment: Instruction for Students

At the end of the session, you should be able to:

- Create a low-tech AAC board appropriate for a patient with _____ to support their EoL communication needs
- Select symbols and words for an AAC board that support EoL connections, reminiscing, and life review
- Choose symbols and words for an AAC board that support basic needs for mealtime, pain management, and toileting

For this assignment, you will create a low-tech AAC board for a client who is near the EoL who has [fill in specific communication disorder]. This patient and family aim to spend quality time together reminiscing about the patient's life, sharing stories and memories. The patient and family also want a way for the patient to indicate thirst, hunger, types of foods they desire, pain or discomfort, and toileting needs.

Your goal is to create an easy-to-navigate board to support the goals the patient's family has identified with a focus on the patient's capacity to identify their needs and interact with the family. The requirements of this board are as follows:

- Between 16 (minimum) and 25 (maximum) stimuli that are personally relevant to the client and family's goals
- A way for your client to indicate affirmatives or negatives, indicate they have a question, and to ask for help

---

Steps to follow:

1. Go to Picto4me—AAC Communi cation Boards for Google Drive https://www.picto4.me/

2. Sign in using your email address.

3. Once your blank communication board is ready, rename it by clicking on "Untitled Board."

---

4. By clicking "Untitled Board," the board editor will pop up. Change the board to 4 columns x 4 rows to allow for at least 16 items (add more as necessary).

5. You can search for pictures by clicking on each square or save your images to your computer and upload them into the board.

6. Once you have completed your board, click the QR code button and this will create a QR code. Scan the code and submit it to the professor within your learning management system or as requested.

REFERENCES

Leslie, P., & Broll, J. (2022). Eating, drinking, and swallowing difficulties: The impacts on, and of, religious beliefs. *Geriatrics (Basel), 7*(2), 41. https://doi.org/10.3390/geriatrics7020041

Pascoe, A., Breen, L. J., & Cocks, N. (2018). What is needed to prepare speech pathologists to work in adult palliative care? *International Journal of Language & Communication Disorders, 53*(3), 542–549.

Pollens, R. (2020). Facilitating client ability to communicate in palliative end-of-life care. *Topics in Language Disorders*, 40(3), 264–277. https://doi.org/10.1097/tld.0000000000000220

Rivers, K. O., Perkins, R. A., & Carson, C. P. (2009). Perceptions of speech-pathology and audiology students concerning death and dying: A preliminary study. *International Journal of Language & Communication Disorders, 44*(1), 98–111.

Stead, A. (2022). End-of-life care for adults. In N. Hall, J. Juengling-Sudkamp, M. L. Gutmann, & E. R. Cohn (Eds.), *Fundamentals in AAC: A case-based approach to enhancing communication.* Plural Publishing.

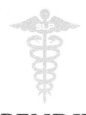

APPENDIX B

End-of-Life Decisional Support Aids for Individuals With Communication or Cognitive Impairments

Michelle Bourgeois and Amanda Stead

DECISION AIDS FOR FACILITATING DECISION MAKING

Decision aids can support patients to indicate their wishes near the end of life (EoL). Strategies that uphold capacity to participate in care decisions are particularly important for patients with communication or cognition impairments or barriers. Communication support strategies effectively support quality of life and decision making in people with progressive neurocognitive disorders (Chang & Bourgeois, 2020; Fried-Oken et al., 2015; Pollens, 2020). Chang and colleagues (2020) demonstrated that decision aids extended a patient's capacity to participate in decisions about their care.

When care decisions are needed, families and health care professionals benefit from understanding the thoughts and preferences of the person who is dying. Even when patients have executed advance care plans, no care plan

can anticipate every possible health scenario, nor can such plans anticipate how people's perspectives and priorities will change with lived experience (see also Chapter 3 and Appendix C). Modified presentation and response options such as visual aids allow patients to demonstrate understanding and reasoning for complex choices (Chang et al., 2020). Speech-language pathologists (SLPs) can serve a vital role as advocates for patients by encouraging use of decision aids. These aids may support comprehension so that patients understand what is happening and may allow some patients to understand the options available and the risks and benefits associated with each option. Evidence has shown that, through these aids, some patients with moderate dementia can demonstrate capacity for EoL decisions.

Below is a series of sample decision aids that SLPs can use to facilitate comprehension, expression, and decision making among patients with impaired communication or cognition.

HOW TO USE A DECISION AID

To use visual decision aids, clinicians must describe the choices and provide visual aids. Clinicians should also provide the risks and benefits (pros and cons) of each choice to facilitate client understanding. Discuss the options thoroughly, along with their pros and cons, using visual aids to accurately inform the client of their options. It is expected that repetition of information will be necessary and beneficial to client comprehension.

Spouses and family members should take part in the discussion. In some cases, loved ones may be able to offer different ways of explaining concepts that are personal to the client. It may be necessary to create new, personalized representations to assist with comprehension and cognition.

Once the client exhibits an adequate understanding of the options and pros and cons, they should be prompted to decide for themselves using their communication board. SLPs and other members of the care team should ensure that neither they nor members of the patient's family are unduly influencing the client. To demonstrate decision-making capacity, the client's decision should be consistent and replicable (see also Chapter 3).

SAMPLE DECISION AIDS

Decision Aid: Participation in Communication of Preference for Burial or Cremation

Patients, family, caregivers, and/or spiritual leaders may engage in discussion about funeral and burial planning. When an individual's preferences are unknown and the patient has communication or cognitive impairments, the SLP may be positioned to support the conversation and thus permit the patient to participate in decision making. Figure B–1 provides an example of a tool with pros and cons associated with burial. Figure B–2 shows an example of a simplified explanation of cremation versus burial with a choice response.

Decision Aid: Client's Preference for Feeding Tube Insertion

Patients with severe medical conditions may be asked their preference related to artificially administered nutrition and hydration. Figure B–3 provides an example of a visual aid to support discussion about the benefits and risks associated with a surgically placed percutaneous endoscopic gastrostomy (PEG) feeding tube.

DECISION AID: CLIENT'S PREFERENCE FOR OTHER ADVANCE CARE PLANNING STEPS

Patients with serious illness, life-limiting conditions, and those nearing the EoL, may be asked their preference about a variety of interventions. For example, do not resuscitate (DNR) or do not intubate (DNI) orders are part of overall advance care planning (Center for Practical Bioethics, 2022; National POLST, 2022). When communication or cognitive barriers exist, SLPs may provide important support to allow the patient to express their preference to forgo specific interventions such as cardiopulmonary resuscitation (CPR), intubation, medication, or terminal sedation. Client-specific visual aids or other communication supports can be created and allow patients to participate in these complex decisions about their care.

Burial

Pros of burial include:

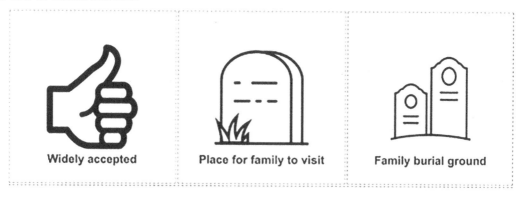

Cons of burial include:

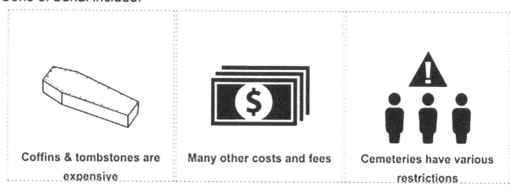

Figure B–1. Example decisional aid to support discussion about the pros and cons of burial.

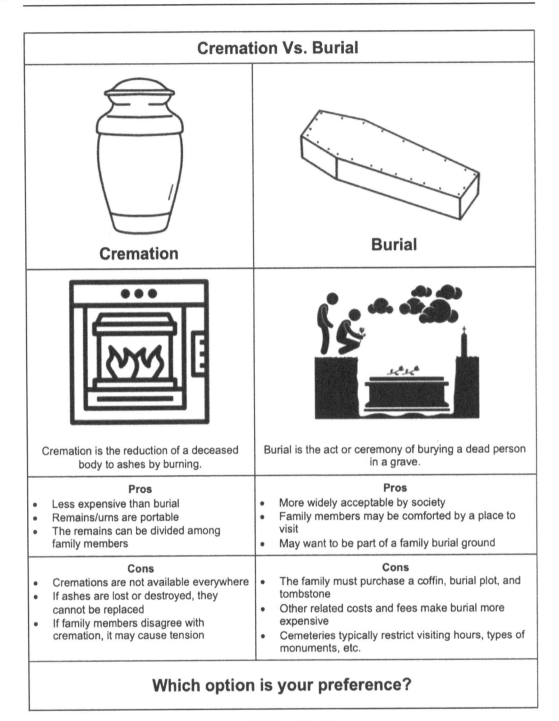

Figure B–2. Example pro and con visual aid for burial preferences.

PEG Tube

Pros of PEG Tube:

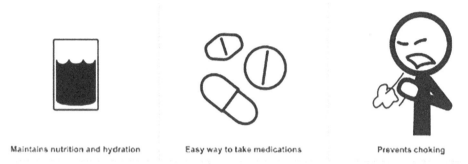

Cons of PEG Tube:

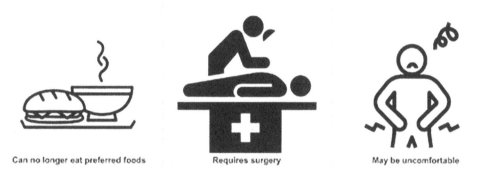

Figure B–3. Example visual aid to support discussion about the risks and benefits of percutaneous endoscopic gastrostomy (PEG) tube placement.

ACKNOWLEDGMENTS

Students at the University of South Florida in the SPA 6564 Seminar in Aging, Cognition, and Communication course partly created these materials. The authors acknowledge the contributions of Brittany Haller, Courtney Solomon, and Shannon Valentine to the development of these examples.

REFERENCES

Center for Practical Bioethics. (2022). *Transportable physician orders for patient preferences (TPOPP)*. https://www.practicalbioethics.org/programs/transportable-physician-orders-for-patient-preferences-tpopp-polst/

Chang, W. Z. D., & Bourgeois, M. S. (2020). Effects of visual aids for end-of-life care on decisional capacity of people with dementia. *American Journal of Speech-Language Pathology, 29*(1), 185–200.

Fried-Oken, M., Mooney, A., & Peters, B. (2015). Supporting communication for patients with neurodegenerative disease. *NeuroRehabilitation, 37*(1), 69–87.

National POLST. (2022). *Honoring the wishes of those with serious illness and frailty.* https://polst.org/

Pollens, R. (2020). Facilitating client ability to communicate in palliative end-of-life care. *Topics in Language Disorders, 40*(3), 264–277. https://doi.org/10.1097/tld.0000000000000220

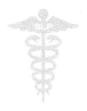

APPENDIX C

Supplemental Reading and Resources

Helen Sharp

In addition to the citations in each chapter, there is a wealth of literature and other resources available to expand your knowledge about death, dying, and end-of-life care. We recognize that this is not a comprehensive list and apologize for oversights. Please help us build resources for SLPs. We welcome your recommendations which can be submitted to Plural Publishing (information@pluralpublishing.com). The content of this appendix is also available on the PluralPlus Companion website and will be updated periodically.

BOOKS

Academic Textbooks

Back, A., Arnold, R, & Tulsky, J. (2009). *Mastering communication with seriously ill patients: Balancing honesty with empathy and hope.* Cambridge University Press.https://doi.org/10.1017/CBO 9780511576454

Bodtke, S. & Ligon, K. (2016). *Hospice and palliative medicine handbook: A clinical guide.* www .hpmhandbook.com

Buckman, R. (1992). *How to break bad news: A guide for health care professionals.* University of Toronto Press.

Cherny, N., Fallow, M. T., Kaasa, S., Portenoy, R. K., & Currow, D. C. (Eds). (2015). *Oxford textbook of palliative medicine* (6th ed). Oxford University Press. https://doi.org/10.1093/med/ 9780198821328.001.0001

Elwyn, G., Edwards, A., & Thompson, R. (Eds.). (2016). *Shared decision making in health care: Achieving evidence-based patient choice.* Oxford University Press. https://doi.org/10.1093/acpr of:oso/9780198723448.001.0001

Ferrell, B. R. (2015). *Pediatric palliative care.* Oxford University Press. https://doi.org/10.10 93/med/9780190244187.001.0001

Macauley, R. C. (2018). *Ethics in palliative care: A complete guide.* Oxford University Press. https://doi.org/10.1093/med/97801993139 45.001.0001

MacDonald, S., Herx, L., & Boyle, A. (Eds.). (2022). *Palliative medicine: A case-based manual* (4th ed). Oxford University Press. https://doi .org/10.1093/oso/9780198837008.001.0001

Wong, A. M. F. (2020). *The art and science of compassion. A primer: Reflections of a physician-chaplain.* Oxford University Press. https://doi .org/10.1093/med/9780197551387.001.0001

Books About Living With a Life-Limiting Condition

Albom, M. (1997). *Tuesdays with Morrie: An old man, a young man, and life's greatest lesson.* Crown.

Bauby, J.-D. (1998). *The diving bell and the butterfly.* Penguin Random House.

Fox, M. J. (2021). *No time like the future: An optimist considers mortality.* Flatiron.

Kalanithi, P. (2017). *When breath becomes air.* Random House.

Mairs, N. (1997). *Waist-high in the world: A life among the nondisabled.* Beacon.

Patchett, A. (2021). *These precious days: Essays.* HarperCollins

Pausch, R. (2012). *The last lecture.* Hyperion.

Popular Press Books About Death, Dying, and End-of-Life Care

Berkowitz, A. (2021). *One by one by one: Making a small difference amid a billion problems.* HarperOne.

Brigham, B. (2022). *Death interrupted: How modern medicine is complicating the way we die.* Walrus Books.

Butler, K. (2019). *The art of dying well: A practical guide to a good end of life.* Scribner.

Clarke, R. (2021). *Dear life: A doctor's story of love, loss, and consolation.* Abacus.

Creagan, E., & Wendel, S. (2018). *Farewell: Vital end-of-life questions with candid answers from a leading palliative and hospice physicians.* Write On Ink Publishing.

Egan, K. (2017). *On living.* Riverhead Books.

Gawande, A. (2014). *Being mortal: Illness, medicine, and what matters in the end.* Picador.

Green, S. (2022). *This is assisted dying: A doctor's story of empowering patients at the end of life.* Scribner.

Lynn, J. (2018). *Handbook for mortals: Guidance for people facing serious illness.* Oxford University Press

Mannix, K. (2018). *With the end in mind: Dying, death, and wisdom in an age of denial.* Little, Brown, Spark.

Marsh, H. (2016). *Do no harm: Stories of life, death, and brain surgery.* Picador.

Miller, B. (2020). *A beginner's guide to the end: Practical advice for living life and facing death.* Simon & Schuster.

Neumann, A. (2016). *The good death: An exploration of dying in America.* Beacon Press.

Nuland, S. B. (1995). *How we die: Reflections of life's final chapter.* Knopf.

Puri, S. (2019). *That good night: Life and medicine in the eleventh hour.* Constable Press.

Sontag, S. (1988). *Illness as metaphor and AIDS and its metaphors.* Picador.

Tisdale, S. (2018). *Advice for future corpses: A practical perspective on death and dying.* Simon & Shuster.

Volandes, A. E. (2015). *The conversation: A revolutionary plan for end-of-life care.* Bloomsbury.

Ware, B. (2019). *The top five regrets of the dying: A life transformed by the dearly departing.* Hay House.

Zitter, J. N. (2017). *Extreme measures: Finding a better path to the end of life.* Avery.

ACADEMIC JOURNALS

- Advances in Palliative Medicine
- American Journal of Hospice and Palliative Medicine
- BMC Palliative Care
- Current Opinion in Supportive and Palliative Care
- Journal of Hospice and Palliative Care
- Journal of Hospice and Palliative Nursing
- Journal of Pain and Symptom Management
- Journal of Palliative Care
- Journal of Palliative Medicine
- OMEGA—Journal of Death and Dying
- Palliative Medicine
- Palliative and Supportive Care

DOCUMENTARIES/MOVIES

- Dying in Your Mother's Arms (Beder, 2022)
- Extremis (Krauss, 2016)
- How to Die in Oregon (Richardson, 2011)
- End Game (Epstein & Friedman, 2018)
- Alternate Endings: 6 New Ways to Die in America (O'Neill & Perri, 2019)
- Griefwalker (Wilson, 2008)
- Dying at Grace (King, 2003)

ASSOCIATIONS FOR HEALTH PROFESSIONALS

- American Academy of Hospice and Palliative Medicine. Website: http://aahpm.org/
- American Geriatrics Society. Website: https://www.americangeriatrics.org/
- Association for Palliative Medicine of Great Britain and Ireland. Website: https://apmonline.org/
- Association for Paediatric Palliative Medicine. Website: https://www.appm .org.uk/
- Canadian Association of MAiD Assessors and Providers (CAMAP). Website: https:// camapcanada.ca/
- Canadian Hospice and Palliative Care Association. Website: https://www.chpca.ca/
- Canadian Network of Palliative Care for Children. Website: https://www.chpca.ca/ projects/canadian-network-of-palliative-care-for-children/
- Hospice Foundation of America. Website: https://hospicefoundation.org/
- International Association for Hospice and Palliative Care (IAHPC). Website: https:// hospicecare.com/home/
- National Association for Hospice at Home (UK). Website: https://www.nahh.org.uk/

- National Institute on Aging. Website: https://www.nia.nih.gov/

COMMUNICATION SKILLS AND PALLIATIVE CARE RESOURCES FOR HEALTH PROFESSIONALS

- Agency for Healthcare Research and Quality (AHRQ). The SHARE approach: A model for shared decision making— Fact sheet. https://www.ahrq.gov/sites/ default/files/publications/files/share-approach_factsheet.pdf
- CAPC-Communication Skills. Training in communication skills to conduct effective goals of care conversations. www .capc.org/training/communication-skills/ clarifying-goals-of-care/
- Five Wishes. Develop communication skills and framing conversations for advance care planning. www.fivewishes .org
- Grenny, J., Patterson, K., McMillan, R., Switzler, A., & Gregory, E. (2021). *Crucial conversations: Tools for talking when the stakes are high* (3rd ed). McGraw Hill.
- Program of Experience in the Palliative Care Approach/Indigenous Program of Experience in the Palliative Care Approach (PEPA/IPEPA). (2020). Learning guide for allied health professionals 2020. https://pepaeducation.com/wp-content/ uploads/2021/01/PEPA_LearningGuide_ AlliedHealthProfessionals_ONLINE.pdf
- Respecting Choices. Training for structured facilitation of advance care planning. www.respectingchoices.org
- VITAL Talk. Online training resources for physicians and other clinicians focused on tools and skills to support goals of care conversations. Website: https://www .vitaltalk.org/

ONLINE RESOURCES TO SUPPORT PATIENTS, FAMILIES, AND CAREGIVERS

- Center for Practical Bioethics. (2022). Caring conversations materials. Available: https://www.practicalbioethics.org/featured-resources/caring-conversations/
- Get Palliative Care. Available: https://getpalliativecare.org/ (English and Spanish Language Resources).
- Hospice Giving Foundation Resources for Families. https://hospicegiving.org/resources/
- Kaiser Family Foundation. (2016). 10 FAQs: Medicare's role in end-of-life care. Available: https://www.kff.org/medicare/fact-sheet/10-faqs-medicares-role-in-end-of-life-care/
- Mannix, K. (2019). *"Dying is not as bad as you think" | BBC Ideas*. Available: https://www.youtube.com/watch?v=CruBRZh8quc
- National POLST Portable Medical Orders. Honoring the wishes of those with serious illness and frailty. Available: https://polst.org/
- Palliative Care Network of Wisconsin. Fast facts and concepts in palliative care. Available: https://www.mypcnow.org/fast-facts/
- The Conversation Project. Tool kits to assist with discussions about preferences for care at the end of life. Available: https://theconversationproject.org/

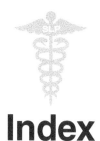

Index

Note: Page numbers in **bold** reference non-text material.

Message banking, **150**, **159**, 165, **166**, **167**, 168, 169
MOLST. *See* Transportable Physician Orders
Morphine. *See* Medication
Mortality. *See* Death
Motor neuron disease, 45, 95, 144 *See also* Amyotrophic Lateral Sclerosis
Motor speech disorders, **104**, **160**, 163, 183–184
Mucopolysaccharidosis, 144
Multidisciplinary team. *See* interdisciplinary team
Multimodal communication, 40, **78**, 98. *See also* Augmentative and alternative communication
Multiple Sclerosis
Muscular dystrophy 118, 144
Music, **16**, 166
  music therapy, **163**, 168

N

National Consensus Project (NCP), 1, **3**, 38
Nasogastric (NG) tube. *See* Tube feeding
Nausea, 14, **17**, **37**, 44, 97, **117**, 119, 122, 128
Neurodiverse, 160
Nonmaleficence. *See* Principles of bioethics
Nonverbal
  patient communication, **103**, **104**, 130, 154, **159**, **163**
  professional communication, **21**, **41**, 48
Noncompliance, 70, 73
Nonspeaking. *See* Nonverbal
Nurse, 2–4, **6**, 22, 24, **25**, 32, 40, 48, 49, **50**, 51, 53, 54, **75**, **78**, 101, 132, 135, 149, 156, **157**, **163–164**
Nursing home, nursing facility. *See* Care setting
Nutrition, 9, 10, **25**, **52**, 110, 115–135, 181–182, 186. *See also* Hydration, Tube feeding

O

Obituary. *See* Personal affairs
Occupational therapy, 2, 4, 24, 47, 149–151
Oncological conditions. *See* Cancer
Opioids. *See* Medication
Oral health, 43, **117**, 119
  dental needs, 120, 133
  dentures, 43

oral care and hygiene, **30**, 36, 43, 48, **50**, 71, **127**, 130–132, 133, 181
Oral intake. *See* Eating
Orientation. *See* Environmental supports
Organ failure, 10–11, 97, 117, 134, 168
Outpatient. *See* Care setting

P

Pain, 1, **3**, 4, 10, 14, **15**, **30**, **44**, 74, 97, 101, 105, 117, 120, 122–123
  communication of, **37**, 49–51, 103, **104**, **109**, 183
  in children, 145–148, 163
Palliative care
  definition of, 1, **3**, 22
Palliative Care Team. *See* Interdisciplinary team
Palliative Performance Scale (PPS), **12**
Partner assisted, **109**, **157–159**, **160**, **163–164**
Paternalism. *See* Parentalism
Patient-centered care, 39
  goals. See Goals, speech-language, Goals of Care
Patient education, **31**, 64, 69, 77, **78**. *See also* Caregiver education, Shared decision making
Parentalism, 64
Payment. *See* Reimbursement
Pediatric 5, 36–37, 43, 81, 85–87, **103**, 141–171, **191**
Percutaneous endoscopic gastrostomy (PEG) tube. *See* Tube feeding
Personal affairs, 4, **37**, **107**
  funeral planning **37**, 51, 53, **107**, 186
Pharmacist, 2, 9, 134, 135
Physical therapy, 4, 24, 149–151, **179**
Physician, 2, **6**, 24, **25**, **50**
  orders. *See* Transportable physician orders
Physician assisted suicide. *See* Medical assistance in dying
Plan of care. *See* Care plan
POLST. *See* Transportable physician orders
Power of attorney for health care. *See* Surrogate decision maker
Primary progressive aphasia. *See* Aphasia
Principles of bioethics. *See* Ethics
Progressive neurological conditions, 10–11, 95–96, 118, 144–145
Proxy. *See* Surrogate decision maker